A Century of Adventure in Northern Health

Phyllis M. Wallace, MPH, CHES
Associate Professor-Allied Health
Ilisagvik College
PO Box 749   Barrow, AK 99723-0749

A Century of Adventure in Northern Health

The Public Health Service
Commissioned Corps in Alaska

1879–1978

Robert Fortuine

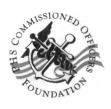

**PHS COMMISSIONED OFFICERS
FOUNDATION** *for the*
Advancement Of Public Health

Landover, MD
2006

ISBN-13: 978-0-9773149-0-4

Printed in the United States of America

♾™ The paper used in this publication meets the minimum requirements
of American National Standard for Information Sciences—Permanence of
Paper for Printed Library Materials, ANSI/NISO Z39.48–1992.

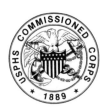

ABOUT THE AUTHOR

Robert Fortuine, MD,CM, MPH, served in the PHS Commissioned Corps for 26 years, 17 of them with the Indian
Health Service in Alaska, where his assignments included
Service Unit Director at the Kanakanak and Bethel hospitals and Director of the Alaska Native Medical Center in
Anchorage. He retired at the rank of captain in 1987, and
since that time has devoted his time mainly to clinical teaching and writing on the history of medicine in northern
regions. He has made his permanent home in the state
since 1963.

This book is respectfully dedicated to the commissioned officers of the U.S. Public Health Service, who have served the people of Alaska with distinction

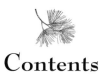

Contents

List of Illustrations

Foreword

he Commissioned Corps of the United States Public Health Service, the oldest and principal health agency of the United States Government, has had a distinguished but largely undocumented history in Alaska. These Public Health Service Commissioned Officers probably have had a greater impact on the health of the people of Alaska than on those of any other region of the United States, in part due to Alaska's federal territorial status from 1867 through 1959, and in part because of the severe and unusual health problems of Alaskans, particularly the Alaska Native peoples.

This book examines the work of the Public Health Service and its predecessor agencies in Alaska from 1879 through 1978—a century of service beginning with the earliest definite record of a Marine-Hospital Service physician in the territory. It details many of the unheralded stories of dedication and selflessness of these health professionals, including service aboard Revenue-Marine cutters and Coast Guard vessels on the Bering Sea Patrol, quarantine services for the control of deadly epidemics, medical care of merchant seamen and fishermen, support to territorial and state health authorities, a major part in the construction of the Alaska Highway, and the provision of direct health care for the Alaska Natives over several generations. A final chapter summarizes important health research carried out in Alaska by the Public Health Service, including some that has been applied on a global scale.

It is noteworthy that many of the officers who served in Alaska chose to remain to serve in private practice or to take up roles in the health agencies of the territorial or state government. One such individual was Erwin Stuart Rabeau, who arrived in Kotzebue in 1946 as 25-year-old commissioned officer and spent the next eleven years in the Arctic, sometimes as the only physician north of Fairbanks. As a result of his medical skills, his travels, and his role in the radio medical traffic, Rabeau became one of the best-known names in northern Alaska. Following several other assignments in Alaska and elsewhere, Rabeau in 1964 became head of the entire Indian Health Service. After 35 years as a PHS Commissioned Officer, he retired in 1981 and returned to Alaska as Director of the State Division of Public Health, a position he held until his death in 1984.

This book, documenting the commitment of Public Health Service Commissioned Officers to the State of Alaska and its people, is published by the Public Health Service Commissioned Officers Foundation for the Advancement of Public Health in collaboration with the University of Alaska Press. The author is Dr. Robert Fortuine, a public health physician who was a commissioned officer with the United States Public Health Service from 1961 until his retirement in 1987. Most of those years were spent in Alaska, where he served at the Alaska Native Hospitals in Kanakanak and Bethel, and at the Alaska Native Medical Center in Anchorage. He has made his permanent home in Alaska since 1963.

The U.S. Public Health Service has a long and proud tradition in Alaska. In a vast territory with sometimes treacherous weather and huge logistical difficulties, and whose diverse peoples have suffered health problems of unprecedented complexity and severity, Commissioned Officers and Civil Service employees of the Public Health Service have brought skill, courage, and enthusiasm to the solution of many difficult problems. Their responsibilities have been great, often at the limits of their training and experience, and they have endured many professional and personal challenges. Those whose endeavors are captured in this book provide the legacy upon which new generations of PHS employees will build. This legacy is one of significant and lasting contributions to the better health of Alaskans. This book will help ensure that the efforts of these earliest health responders will not be forgotten, as we stand on their shoulders and, with continued spirit, determination, and zeal, reach for excellence in public health practice throughout the world.

Richard H. Carmona

Richard H. Carmona, M.D., M.P.H., F.A.C.S.
Vice Admiral, USPHS
United States Surgeon General

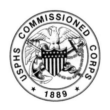

Preface

Recognition of the need for a national public health focus dates back to 1798 when Congress established the Marine-Hospital Service to provide medical services to merchant seamen. That was the beginning of the US Public Health Service and remains a date emblazoned on its seal.

The need for a specialized cadre of professionals dedicated to public health was recognized in 1871 when President Grant appointed Dr. John Woodworth as the first Surgeon General of the United States. Woodward, a hero of the Union Army in the Civil War, set up a new personnel system along military lines, a characteristic that today gives the Commissioned Corps its unique readiness characteristic. The PHS Commissioned Corps was formally authorized by Congress on January 4, 1889. Initially restricted to physicians, the Commissioned Corps evolved into a uniformed service representing all of the major health disciplines.

In its formative years, the Corps devoted its resources to health issues of the day, including care for merchant seamen, prevention of communicable diseases, and improvements in sanitation and environmental conditions. As the Corps' responsibilities have broadened, officers have been instrumental in pioneering research and applications in bacteriology, virology, parasitology, epidemiology, and nutritional diseases.

Corps officers played vital roles in both World Wars and the Korean conflict, during which the President placed the Corps in military status. Many officers also served in the Vietnam War. PHS officers are currently detailed to the areas of conflict including Kosovo, Afghanistan, and Iraq to provide public health and medical expertise. Hundreds of officers served to provide emergency services at all three sites resulting from the terrorist acts of September 11, 2001, as well as during the anthrax crisis of late 2001. A large group of officers also provided services to the victims of the December 2004 Asian tsunami. In the wake of the devastating hurricanes to hit the US Gulf Coast in 2005, fully one third of all corps officers were deployed to provide needed health and medical assistance to those communities.

Today the Corps serves all health agencies of the Department of Health and Human Services, including CDC, NIH, FDA, and the Indian Health Service, as well as providing all of the health and medical services for the US Coast Guard and the Federal Bureau of Prisons. Officers are detailed to many other federal agencies such as the EPA, the Department of Justice, the State Department, and, of course, the Department of Defense. The more than 6,000 officers of the Corps serve in every state in our nation and 550 locations worldwide.

The PHS Commissioned Corps is one of seven uniformed services whose members are on duty 24 hours a day to respond to national needs. The Corps' mission is "To protect and to advance the health and safety of our nation."

The history of the Public Health Service in Alaska dates back to 1879. That record includes early contributions to establish basic medical service to the developing territory and a remarkable history of providing a broad health and environmental program serving the Alaska Natives. Along the way, officers on active duty and retired from the Commissioned Corps have taken a leadership role in the staffing of state and local health departments as well as the private sector of medicine throughout the early territorial days and, since 1959, to the State of Alaska.

This monograph describing the seminal role of PHS Commissioned Officers in the shaping of the health status of the citizens of Alaska is a true record of "Service with Distinction." It is intended to serve not only as a valuable reference of a dedicated commitment of selfless health professionals to that broad multi-ethnic community, but it also has the potential for use as a model in many other broad health programs serving the wide global community.

One of that dedicated band of health professionals is the present work's author, Dr. Robert Fortuine, who has devoted nearly his entire professional career to the enhancement of the health of the Alaska Native people, and, following his retirement, to documenting the history of health and health services in northern regions.

This book was produced as an educational effort of the PHS Commissioned Officers Foundation for the Advancement of Public Health. The Foundation, a nonprofit affiliate of the PHS Commissioned Officers Association, supports broad public and professional educational efforts in the field of public health.

Jerrold M. Michael

Rear Admiral (Ret.) Jerrold M. Michael
President, PHS Commissioned Officers Foundation
for the Advancement of Public Health

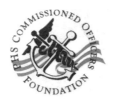

Acknowledgments

his monograph traces its origin to the invitation by Captain Jay Butler, then director of the CDC Arctic Investigations Program in Anchorage, Alaska, for me to present a paper on the history of the Public Health Service in Alaska during the national meeting of the PHS Commissioned Officers Association to be held in May 2004 in Anchorage. Following the meeting, Rear Admiral (Ret.) Jerrold M. Michael suggested that the presentation be expanded and documented for publication by the PHS Commissioned Officers Foundation for the Advancement of Public Health. I am particularly indebted to Rear Admiral Michael for his constant encouragement and enthusiasm in seeing this project through to its conclusion, and to the members of the board of directors and the staff of the foundation for their support of this undertaking. Captain (Ret.) Gerard Farrell, Executive Director of the Commissioned Officers Association, has been helpful in many ways. Dr. Alexandra Lord of the Office of the PHS Historian greatly assisted my research by making available documentary materials from Washington.

A special measure of appreciation must go to Captain (Ret.) Milton Z. Nichaman, who contributed countless hours of his time to editing the manuscript. His many suggestions and comments have greatly improved the final text. He was also kind enough to make a trip to Alaska to oversee the final details of the publication process.

I would like to offer sincere thanks and recognition to the following individuals for their financial support for the printing of this monograph: Rear Admiral (Ret.) John W. Cashman, Rear Admiral (Ret.) Clifford Cole, Rear Admiral

(Ret.) Emery A. Johnson (now deceased), Rear Admiral (Ret.) Jerrold M. Michael, Captain (Ret.) Milton Z. Nichaman, Mrs. Mary Ann Rabeau, Mrs. Nancy Rabeau-Lovering, Captain (Ret.) Jack C. Robertson, Rear Admiral (Ret.) John G. Todd, Rear Admiral (Ret.) John J. Walsh, and Mrs. Doris D. Wherritt (now deceased).

In preparing this history, I was reminded of the many PHS colleagues and friends with whom I have worked in Alaska over a span of 29 years. My special mentors included E. S. ("Stu") Rabeau, who, in 1962, was the Area Director in the Aberdeen Area of the Division of Indian Health. Already an Alaska legend for his many years as virtually the sole physician in northern Alaska, Stu promised me an assignment in Alaska if I would remain in the PHS beyond my two-year draft commitment. I jumped at the chance. When I arrived in Alaska at the Anchorage airport in June 1963 with my wife, Sheila, one-year-old daughter, and a large German shepherd dog, I was personally welcomed by Kazumi Kasuga. Holman R. Wherritt, formerly of the Aberdeen Area, had come to Alaska the previous year and soon became the Alaska Area Director. He was my immediate superior throughout my four "bush" years in Kanakanak and Bethel, and I later worked for him a third time while a resident in IHS headquarters in 1968–1969. After four *Wanderjahre* for training and an assignment on the Navajo Reservation, I returned to Alaska in 1971 as Director of the Alaska Native Medical Center, succeeding Martha Wilson, who had ably led the hospital for eight years during its transition from tuberculosis sanatorium to referral hospital. The Area Director at that time was John Lee, who was steering the program through a time of great change. All of these, sadly, have now passed on. Each had special strengths, but a common thread was their respect and commitment to involving the Alaska Natives in a meaningful way in their own health program. Each taught me and guided me through many difficult situations.

Some of my clinical colleagues and closest friends over the years should also be mentioned, since they have especially brightened my outlook and lent me help and support on countless occasions. Space does not permit a full listing, but I must name at least David Dolese and Charles H. Neilson (both deceased), M. Walter Johnson, David W. Templin, George Brenneman, Gloria K. Park, Daniel J. O'Connell, Douglas Smole, and Thomas S. Nighswander. To these especially, and to all my other friends in the PHS over the years, I offer special thanks and good wishes.

I would like to express my deepest thanks to Erica Hill and her staff at the University of Alaska Press for their outstanding work and cooperation in the design and production of this book.

Robert Fortuine
Wasilla, Alaska

Chapter 1
Background

T he United States Public Health Service, the oldest and principal health agency of the United States Government, has had a distinguished but largely undocumented history in Alaska. In the three published histories of the service there is only cursory mention of Alaska, usually within the context of some larger health issue.[1] Yet, the Public Health Service probably has had a greater impact on the health of the people of Alaska than it has had on those of any other region of the United States, in part due to Alaska's federal territorial status from 1867 through 1959, and in part because of the unusual and severe health problems of Alaskans, particularly the Alaska Native[2] peoples. Moreover, since these health problems occurred in a land with a harsh climate and difficult logistical issues of supply and transportation, they have required a unique set of creative solutions.

In this account I will examine the work of the PHS (and its predecessor agencies) in Alaska from 1879 through 1978—a century of service beginning with the earliest definite record of the Marine-Hospital Service in the territory. This record will be examined under seven general headings: 1) service at sea with the Revenue-Cutter Service and the Coast Guard; 2) marine hospital services for the medical care of merchant seamen and other beneficiaries; 3) quarantine, disease control, and general public health support to the Alaska territorial and state governments; 4) World War II and its aftermath; 5) support to the Alaska

Native health programs of the Bureau of Education and the Bureau of Indian Affairs; 6) the work of the Division of Indian Health (later the Indian Health Service); and 7) health research in northern climes.

Although each administrative unit of the Public Health Service had a primary mission, services inevitably overlapped, especially since officers were often called upon to respond to situations beyond the limits of their assigned responsibilities. I have organized this book largely by agency or function rather than by a straight chronological approach, to avoid confusion and to help the reader appreciate the diverse ways that the Public Health Service has assisted Alaska to confront its health problems.

Alaska and Its People

Alaska's 591,000 square miles are equivalent to about one fifth the size of the continental United States. The outer limits of Alaska, when superimposed on the map of these states, reach from San Diego to Atlanta to Duluth.

The major physical features of the state include the great central Alaska Range including Mt. McKinley, the Brooks Range in the north, the southeastern Chugach-Wrangells Range and the volcanic Aleutian Range extending westward across the northern Pacific. The great rivers include the mighty Yukon, with its main tributaries the Tanana and the Koyukuk, the Kuskokwim, the Nushugak, the Noatak, the Copper, and the Susitna. Much of the land mass in the western and northern coastal regions is low-lying marshy tundra, whereas the interior has upland taiga and Southeast Alaska still has rain forests of majestic evergreens. The islands of the Pacific and Bering Sea are treeless, windswept volcanic outcroppings of rock and grasses.

Alaska has not one, but three climates. The Panhandle, the Pacific Rim, Kodiak Island, the Alaska Peninsula, and the Aleutians have a maritime climate with relatively mild temperatures, fogs, heavy precipitation, and frequent and

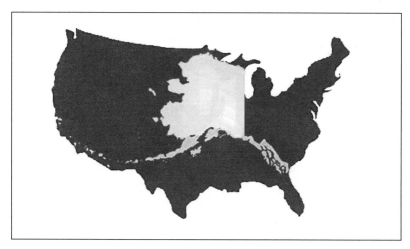

Figure 1. Map of Alaska superimposed on map of the continental United States. *Public domain*

unpredictable storms. North and west of the Brooks Range the climate is typically arctic with very low temperatures, little snowfall, and short, cool summers. The interior climate is continental and characterized by warm summer temperatures and extremely cold winter temperatures.

The population of Alaska, according to 2003 Census estimates, is about 648,000, with 42 percent of those living in Anchorage. Nearly 30 percent of the population lives in the rural areas, known locally in Alaska as the "bush." Alaska Natives, including Eskimos, Indians, and Aleuts, account for almost 20 percent of the population, and about half of those live in the remote roadless areas of Alaska in the interior, northern and western coastal areas, Kodiak Island, Alaska Peninsula, and the Aleutian Islands. These indigenous peoples are thought to have migrated from Eastern Asia over the Bering Land Bridge 10,000 to 15,000 years ago. Many went south, but others stayed to eke out a remarkable existence in this forbidding land. Alaska Natives have a rich mosaic of languages and cultures. Eskimo cultures predominate in the western and northern coastal regions, the Alaska Peninsula, and the Pacific Rim,

Indians occupy the Interior and the Panhandle, and Aleuts inhabit the Aleutian and Pribilof Islands. The first Europeans to reach Alaska were Russians, in the early eighteenth century. There were many Russian voyages for the purpose of exploration and sea-mammal hunting along Alaskan coasts during the latter half of that century, along with major expeditions or trading voyages by the English, French, Spanish, and Americans. In the late eighteenth century the Russians established a few permanent settlements, including those at Unalaska, Three Saints' Bay on Kodiak Island, and New Archangel (now Sitka). In 1799 several Russian fur-trading companies were amalgamated into the Russian-American Company, which established its capital at Sitka.

In 1867 the United States, largely in an attempt to forestall British expansion, purchased Alaska from Russia for $7.2 million dollars. The new territory, known derisively as "Seward's Icebox" or "Walrussia," was administered first by the army and then by the navy until the first primitive civil government was established by Congress in 1884. After years of relative neglect, Alaska was suddenly put on the map again with the discovery of Klondike gold in 1897, when the territory became the staging area for hopeful prospectors heading for the Yukon Territory by trudging over White Pass and Chilkoot Trails or by boating up the great rivers. Over the next few decades other gold rushes occurred, notably at Nome in 1900 and at Fairbanks a few years later.

Over the next 40 years Alaska was rarely noticed nationally until the occasion of the race to Nome with diphtheria antitoxin in the winter of 1925. Although this was a rather small epidemic, as Alaskan epidemics go, it intruded on the national consciousness with much media hype, even leading to the placement of a bronze sculpture of the sled dog Balto in New York's Central Park. Commemoration of this feat played a part in the establishment, in 1972, of the Iditarod sled dog race from Anchorage to Nome.

In the decades leading up to the Second World War, Alaska was mercilessly exploited by outside industrial interests, especially the salmon canning industry and the great mining and timber conglomerates. The war itself brought new recognition to Alaska because of its strategic location and natural resources. The Japanese not only bombed military bases in Alaska, but invaded and briefly held two American islands, Attu and Kiska, in the Aleutians. The war also brought the construction of the Alcan Highway (now the Alaska Highway) and a huge influx of new residents, both military and civilian, to build bases and provide support services to the troops.

Following the war many workers and veterans stayed on, and Alaska's economy began to grow and diversify, this time based largely on Cold War military spending. In 1959 Alaska became the 49th state and for the first time had an elected governor, two US Senators and a Representative, and withal the opportunity to set its own course. Since statehood the political system has had its ups and downs, sometimes with a faintly comic opera quality, but Alaskans have made their political mark through important and strong national political heavyweights such as Senator Ernest Gruening in the 1960s and Senator Ted Stevens, recently Chair of the Senate Appropriations Committee.

The greatest earthquake ever recorded in North America—9.2 on the Richter scale—occurred in Alaska on Good Friday, March 27, 1964. Loss of life was blessedly light, but the changes to the landscape were enormous. The city of Anchorage suffered severe damage, and the largest PHS facility in the state, the Alaska Native Hospital in Anchorage, had a close call. Some communities in Prince William Sound and on Kodiak Island were inundated and destroyed by tsunamis and were forced to relocate.

Large deposits of petroleum were discovered in 1968 in Prudhoe Bay, on the North Slope of Alaska east of Barrow. Since that time politics, influence peddling, budgets, tax policy, degradation of the environment, and even Alaskan personal income have been dominated in some form or other by oil. In 1971 Congress passed the historic Alaska Native Claims Settlement Act, giving Alaska Natives a cash settlement of nearly $1 billion and title to about 44 million acres of land. Under its terms Natives in Alaska organized into twelve regional for-profit and twelve nonprofit corporations. With the question of land title settled, a consortium of large industrial corporations built the 800-mile Trans-Alaska Pipeline from Prudhoe Bay to Valdez in the period 1974–1977.

In the 1970s the Alaska State Legislature wisely created the Alaska Permanent Fund by putting aside a portion of the state's oil royalties into a trust, which now totals over $33 billion. Since 1982 some of the earnings from this fund have been paid out annually to individual Alaskans, in amounts ranging up to $1,800. Much political maneuvering in Alaska relates to the extent that the income from this fund should be used to support state government, which at present is almost totally dependent on royalties from oil production.

On Good Friday, March 24, 1989, twenty-five years after the 1964 earthquake, the supertanker *Exxon Valdez* ploughed into Bligh Reef in Prince William Sound, spilling a large amount of oil that caused severe environmental damage to wildlife and commercial fisheries, some of the effects of which are still apparent.

Alaska remains in the news today for yet another oil-related story—the question of petroleum exploration and drilling in the Arctic National Wildlife Refuge, or ANWR. Major political forces are lined up on both sides of this issue, and the story of this titanic struggle between conservationists and the resource developers remains to be played out on the national scene.[3]

An Overview of Health History in Alaska

Paleopathological examination of frozen bodies and mummies from Alaska has provided a wealth of historical information on health before Westerners arrived in Alaska, and has made it possible to identify several types of serious infections among the people, almost certainly including tuberculosis, as well as the occurrence of various parasites, arthritis, and other chronic diseases. Early explorers found a population with many serious diseases and disabilities, including eye and ear disease, missing limbs, congenital malformations, and milder infections, especially of the skin. Explorers, traders, and early missionaries also discovered complex healing systems in each culture. Shamans employed magico-religious techniques, whereas empirical healers made use of healing plant and animal substances and sophisticated surgical techniques.

Ships' surgeons provided the earliest Western-style medical care in Alaska, mainly to their shipmates and to colonists, but also sometimes to the Alaska Natives. The Russians stationed the first resident physician in their capital at Sitka in 1820 and maintained a well-equipped hospital there until the American purchase. They also made wide use of so-called *feldshers*, a kind of physician assistant, many of whom were Alaska Natives who were trained in Alaska.

After the American purchase, the quality and availability of medical care diminished almost immediately. For the remainder of the nineteenth century, the only physicians in the territory were a few from the army and navy, one or two enterprising private practitioners in Sitka, Skagway, Dyea, Nome, and Juneau, a few scattered missionary physicians, and the physicians of the Marine-Hospital Service.

Health conditions in the eighteenth and nineteenth centuries were bad and getting worse. Deadly epidemic diseases, including smallpox, influenza, mumps, measles, diphtheria, scarlet fever, and pertussis, were introduced and exacted a fearful toll among the Alaska Natives. The most damaging of these were a great smallpox epidemic in 1835–1840 and a devastating epidemic of influenza and measles in 1900. Tuberculosis and sexually transmitted diseases were also widespread and increasing, especially among Alaska Natives. The pernicious effects of alcohol and tobacco, both introduced by Europeans and embraced by the Natives, also caused serious health problems.[4]

After 1885 the Bureau of Education, a federal agency of the Interior Department, operated a system of village schools in Alaska. Since teachers repeatedly reported that the children had many serious health problems, the agency by 1907 had begun to hire physicians and nurses, initially as teachers but later as full-time health workers. It had opened some makeshift hospitals for the Alaska Natives, first in a rented building in Juneau in 1910 and later in existing school buildings around the territory. Budgets were very tight and the facilities were few and poorly equipped. The health program gradually grew, however, with emphasis on prevention (then called "hygiene") and the isolation of the sick. New hospitals were built at Juneau, Akiak, and Noorvik, and for several summers the Bureau operated a health boat—the *Martha Angeline*—to serve the isolated villages on the Yukon River.

The most important problems of this era were overwhelmingly infectious diseases, particularly tuberculosis, but also epidemic diseases such as influenza, measles, scarlet fever, diphtheria, and pertussis. The deadly worldwide Spanish Flu epidemic was brought to Alaska in two waves, by the last ships in the fall of 1918 and again from the first ships in the spring of 1919, both times causing a high mortality.

In March 1931 the health program of the Bureau of Education was turned over to the Bureau of Indian Affairs (BIA), thus bringing Alaska in line with the health services for Native Americans in the rest of the country. During this era the bureau (later known as the Alaska Native Service, or ANS) built new hospitals at Mountain Village, Kotzebue, Unalaska, Bethel, Kanakanak, and Tanana, while expanding programs, especially in public health nursing and dental care.

Shortly after passage of the Social Security Act in 1935, the territorial government organized a de facto health department under a part-time commissioner to serve as a conduit for receiving grants from the Social Security Administration, Children's Bureau, and Public Health Service. The new department concentrated its efforts on communicable disease control and environmental safety.

The exigencies and shortages of World War II, however, led to significant cutbacks in health services for Alaska Natives, as many physicians and nurses joined the military services or took up other assignments related to the war effort. One of the direct casualties of the war was the Bureau of Indian Affairs hospital at Unalaska, which was destroyed during the Japanese attack on Dutch Harbor in June 1942.

After the war the Alaska State Legislature authorized, for the first time, a formal Alaska Department of Health (ADH), a board of health, and a full-time commissioner of health. The new department, together with the Bureau of Indian Affairs, launched as its first priority a comprehensive attack on tuberculosis, then the principal killer of Alaska Natives, with mortality, incidence, and infection rates among the highest ever recorded anywhere.

One of the principal strategies for both ADH and BIA was to obtain surplus military hospitals and their equipment and to convert them into sanatoria. The first, in 1945, became a BIA facility at Skagway, followed by a territorial sanatorium at Seward in 1946, and a combined BIA/ADH orthopedic hospital and BIA sanatorium the following year at Sitka, the latter two forming the Mt. Edgecumbe Medical Center. Around the same time, Congress passed appropriations for two large new sanatoria, one at Mt. Edgecumbe, which opened in 1950, and one in Anchorage, which began operations in 1953. The following year a large new field hospital at Bethel replaced the original facility that had burned in 1950. The ADH also converted military surplus ships and vehicles, including a railway car, into mobile health units, each of which carried a physician, a public health nurse, and an x-ray survey unit. The assault on tuberculosis also included a tuberculosis registry, massive tuberculin testing and x-ray surveys, and the widespread use of the antituberculosis vaccine BCG.

At the peak of the tuberculosis campaign in 1956, some 1,398 Alaskans were hospitalized either in Alaska or in Seattle. Over 90 percent were Alaska Natives, amounting to about one out of every 28 Natives in the territory. Then, in the mid-1950s and into the 1960s, a series of studies were carried out in Alaska on the use of home treatment with new antituberculosis drugs and the use of the drug isoniazid INH as a prophylactic regimen. These programs were successful beyond all expectations and soon led to the virtual emptying of the system of sanatoria so laboriously built up over the previous two decades. By 1968 not a single tuberculosis death was recorded in Alaska.[5]

The emptying of the tuberculosis hospitals led to increased attention being paid to many other health problems, including other infectious diseases, dental disease, some emerging chronic disorders, mental health, and to the whole neglected area of village sanitation. In 1965, the 400-bed tuberculosis sanatorium at Anchorage finally officially became the Alaska Native Medical Center (ANMC), a general referral hospital for all Alaska Natives. On a smaller scale, the Mt. Edgecumbe Hospital also became a general medical and surgical facility.[6]

The private medical sector in Alaska developed in a similar fashion to the profession in other American frontier territories and states. The first physicians came as adventurers shortly after the purchase and settled in Sitka, the old Russian capital. In the latter part of the nineteenth century, a bevy of physicians came, first to Juneau, and later to Skagway and Dyea, either as gold prospectors and miners themselves, or to profit from the great influx of people who came to Southeast Alaska en route to the Klondike. As gold was discovered in other areas, such as Rampart, Nome, and Fairbanks, other physicians came north and a few stayed on, almost all of them in the larger, predominantly non-Native communities. A few supplemented their income by contracting with the Marine-Hospital Service, the Bureau of Education, and the Bureau of Indian Affairs.

Most nonfederal Alaskan hospitals began as mission hospitals, although later they became staffed primarily by private physicians. As Alaskan commercial interests grew, especially mining, salmon canning, timber production, and the Alaska Railroad, companies either hired physicians or contracted with them to care for the workers.

The larger towns, notably Anchorage, Fairbanks, Juneau, Ketchikan, Cordova, and Seward, grew rapidly in the years leading up to World War II, when there was a large influx of military construction workers. These boom conditions largely continued after the war, leading to new hospital construction and an influx of more physicians and other health workers. Many former military physicians (and later PHS physicians) opted to remain in Alaska after their term of service was completed. Most specialists tended to concentrate in Anchorage and Fairbanks, which became referral centers for other areas of the territory.

Chapter 2
At Sea with the Revenue-Cutter Service and the Coast Guard

The United States Marine-Hospital Service (MHS) was established in 1798 principally to provide medical care to merchant seamen in US port cities, with the hospitals financed by a salary deduction from the pay of each sailor. The following year, personnel of the Revenue-Marine Service (RMS), which had been established in 1789, became eligible for care under a similar financial arrangement. The principal functions of the RMS were to ensure that tariffs were not avoided, to protect shipping from unlawful interdiction, and to intercept contraband, notably liquor. Both the MHS and the RMS were located administratively in the Treasury Department and worked closely together from their inception. The MHS sometimes assigned physicians to cutters to provide medical care to the crew and to merchant seamen, act as quarantine officers, and carry out other health functions. The Revenue-Marine Service became officially known as the Revenue-Cutter Service in 1863.

In Alaska, however, the job was much more complicated. The officers and crews of the cutters had the added duties of enforcing all US laws, carrying out hydrographic surveys, and protecting the Pribilof fur-seal herd from pelagic sealing. Cutters were also engaged in exploration, search and rescue, and the transportation of officials, criminals, and the sick from one place to another. For nearly the entire decade of the 1890s, cutters even regularly ferried reindeer from Siberia to Alaska.

The first revenue cutter to visit Alaska was the *Lincoln*, sailing from San Francisco in July 1867 with Captain W. A. Howard in command. The ship carried a surgeon, but we have no information regarding his name or whether he was indeed from the Marine-Hospital Service.[1] The following year the cutter *Wayanda* cruised from the southern tip of Alaska to the Bering Sea with Dr. Thomas T. Minor aboard. His principal function, however, appeared to be to collect natural history specimens for the Smithsonian Institution and evaluate the territory's resources.[2]

The first cutter known to carry a Marine-Hospital Service physician in Alaskan waters was the *Richard Rush*, which was commissioned in 1879 for a patrol voyage to the Gulf of Alaska and Bering Sea.[3] Among the regular duties of its men were exploration, guarding the US sea frontier, rescuing shipwrecked sailors, overseeing the whaling fleet, collecting customs, and enforcing the law, plus a new function—the provision of medical care to sailors of the commercial whaling and fishing fleets, and to Alaska Natives living in remote coastal villages.

The medical officer aboard the *Rush* in 1879 was Robert White, described as "Assistant Surgeon, United States Marine-Hospital Service."[4] White wrote a detailed account

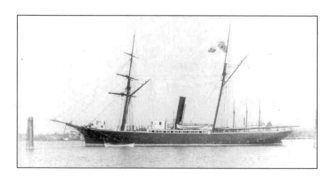

Figure 2. US Revenue Cutter *Richard Rush* around 1875. *USCG Photo*

of his medical activities, modestly called "Notes," as an appendix to Captain Bailey's extensive report on conditions in Alaska.[5] He began his account as follows:

> In addition to the discharge of the duties of medical officer of the vessel, with the concurrence of the commanding officer, professional assistance and medicines were furnished to the inhabitants of the various settlements at which the steamer touched during the cruise. These services were extensively required, as at most of the points in question the natives and whites alike are without medical attendance of any kind other than such as is furnished by the native Indian physicians or "shamans."[6]

The cutter first visited many of the Tlingit villages of Southeast Alaska, where White noted a high prevalence of sexually transmitted diseases, tuberculosis, rheumatism, and the adverse effects of tobacco and alcohol. He also described, in some detail, the traditional healing methods of the Alaska Natives, including their use of plants, shamanic ceremonies, methods of childbirth and newborn care, and burial practices.

The *Rush* next sailed across the Gulf of Alaska to Kodiak, and thence down the Aleutian Chain. Again White observed many sexually transmitted diseases, widespread tuberculosis, and the results of recent severe measles epidemics that had caused a high mortality among the Aleuts. The cutter then proceeded to the Pribilof Islands, far out in the Bering Sea, where White was posted for two months while the ship went farther north with another medical officer.

White's report is measured and low key, but it is apparent that he was having a good time and was fascinated by the sights, sounds, and smells of the voyage. He was clearly sympathetic toward the plight of the Alaska Natives and made a serious effort to identify the cultural implications of their health status.[7]

From 1880 on, at least one cutter made an annual trip through the stormy Bering Sea when ice conditions permitted, usually into the Arctic Ocean as far north as Barrow, a cruise which became known as the Bering Sea Patrol. The majority of these ships carried a medical officer of the Marine-Hospital Service. A surgeon was on board the cutter *Thomas Corwin* on the first of these cruises in 1880 under the command of Captain C. L. Hooper, but the surgeon is not mentioned by name. Hooper related in his official report that when he was walking around the village of Point Barrow accompanied by his surgeon, he heard of a sick man then being treated by a shaman for "evil spirits." The captain told the Eskimos that his medical officer was himself a kind of shaman and asked them whether he could consult on the case. After some persuasion it was agreed that the surgeon could go as far as the entrance to the tent and the patient would be brought to see him there. The individual was found to be suffering from paralysis of the left side and a skin disease. The surgeon left some medicine which the patient was probably not allowed to take.[8]

The next MHS physician to reach arctic waters was Irving Rosse, who sailed in the summer of 1881 on the *Corwin*, now under command of the redoubtable Captain Michael ("Roaring Mike") Healy, one of the most compelling characters in Alaskan history.[9] The ship, which also carried naturalist John Muir and the great ethnologist Edward W. Nelson, spent considerable time in both the Bering Sea and the Arctic Ocean, even visiting remote Wrangel Island, north of Siberia. A valuable part of Rosse's report is his description of the St. Lawrence Islanders a few years after a disastrous famine there. Although said to be most genial in person, his writings betray a measure of pretension and pompousness. After a discourse on the value of alcohol for arctic explorers, for example, Rosse wrote:

> Illicit traders, taking advantage of this northern craving
> for drink, have of late years been in the habit of supplying the most villainous compounds, in exchange for small
> quantities of which the improvident Eskimo gives his

choicest furs. Some captured specimens of these prohib-
ited articles . . . proved on examination to be nothing but
cheap alcohol of a highly inflammable nature to which a
little coloring matter had been added. Loath as I am to
give the least encouragement to intemperance, being
rather an advocate of temperance, I cannot help thinking
that it would be a step in the right direction, and one
productive of good, if instead of the present prohibitory
measures the fur companies were allowed to sell small
quantities of beer and claret. In addition to their value as
antiscorbutics, their use would be eminently better for
the natives from a moral point of view than the present
use of "quass," a vile native decoction made from sugar
and flour, both of which articles the traders have a right
to dispose of in unlimited quantities.[10]

Other topics of interest to Rosse included eye disease,
the effects of arctic conditions on disease, wound healing
under arctic conditions, and the monstrous Alaskan mosquitoes:

Mosquitoes were found to be quite troublesome at Saint
Michael's. How strange that the busy drones of these little
dipterous insects, recalling the solicitations for a *pour boire*
in a French café, should opportune one's ears at a spot so
far north beyond the domain of the ordinary "globe trot-
ter" and unknown to tourists! . . . [A]n instance is even
recorded of their affording material for Eskimo wit at
Lieutenant Schwatka's expense, who was facetiously
styled by these people "the big mosquito."[11]

Other physicians accompanied cutters on their northern cruises in these years, and as early as 1885 Captain Healy
paid special tribute to the physicians of the Marine-
Hospital Service who had sailed with him:

The value of the services of a medical officer in the Arctic
cannot be too highly estimated, the attendance on the
officers and crew of the *Corwin* forming but a small portion of the duty which he is called on to perform. . . . The
crews of the [whaling] fleet comprise upwards of one

thousand men, and a large percentage of these are annually treated by the medical officer of the *Corwin*. . . . When
the *Corwin* first went north the Indians had a great re-
pugnance to receiving medical attendance from a doctor,
but would resort to their shaman to cure all their ailments.
Now, however, the doctor is sought by them in all their
ills, and their faith in his power is truly surprising.[12]

In 1886 the revenue cutter *Bear*, the most distinguished
and beloved of Alaskan ships, was sent north for the first
of over 40 annual cruises. The next year Dr. W. D. Bratton
of the Marine-Hospital Service was the first of a long series
of physicians to serve on the ship. Among the 222 patients
he examined in 1887, many of them Alaska Natives, there
were nine cases of rheumatic fever, four cases of pulmonary tuberculosis, and two cases of scrofula. Local injuries,
skin diseases, constipation, nasal catarrh, neuralgia, and
acute bronchitis were the commonest illnesses reported. An
Alaska Native young adult, presumably transported by the
Bear, died of measles and liver failure at the MHS Hospital
in San Francisco and his remains were autopsied.[13]

Assistant Surgeon C. H. Gardner, the medical officer on
the cutter *Rush* in 1892, reported that during his cruise in
the Bering Sea he treated 18 cases on the ship and another

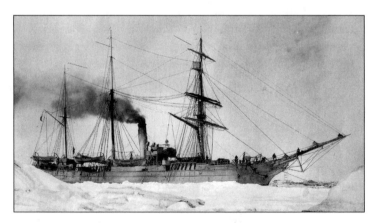

Figure 3. US Revenue Cutter *Bear*, with the *Thomas Corwin* in the background. *USCG Photo*

35 on other ships or ashore, adding that 15 of them, probably Alaska Natives, were not entitled to care under MHS regulations. Other eligible seamen, he noted, were treated by medical officers of naval vessels in the region. The captain, in his report, stated that Dr. Gardner had also performed several surgical operations and had provided medical assistance at all the villages where the vessel called.[14]

The medical officer on the 1895 voyage of the *Rush* was Assistant Surgeon J. H. Oakley. The vessel spent most of the summer in the southern waters of the Gulf of Alaska, the Aleutians, and the Pribilofs. His duties, besides those on his own ship, included medical care for seamen on 13 American and four British ships. Rumors of smallpox aboard a British sealer fortunately proved to be false following an investigation. Oakley treated Alaska Natives ashore in five villages in Prince William Sound and the Aleutians, noting their prevailing diseases to be scrofula, tuberculosis, and syphilis.[15]

During the *Bear's* 1891 cruise, Healy heard of a stranded whaler who had spent the winter in a tiny shanty near Point Hope and sent his surgeon, Dr. Samuel J. Call, who had joined the cutter service that year, to investigate.[16] Call reported back:

> I accompanied the whalers to their station, distant about ten miles, where I found the patient in a most pitiable condition. He was lying on a rickety bunk in a small, dirty room. His clothing consisted of a deerskin covering for the extremities and a shirt for the body. The shirt had been worn continuously for almost four months. His finger nails were from a quarter inch to a half inch in length. Vermin covered his body. The man's left foot, almost to the heel, was a mass of distorted, foul-smelling, gangrenous tissue. Three fingers of the left hand were mere stubs. I find it necessary to amputate his left leg and three fingers of his left hand. These operations will seriously endanger his life. . . . The patient has been informed of

his condition and has consented to the operation, knowing that he may not survive it, and that it is his only chance for life.[17]

The patient did indeed survive and returned south with the *Bear* that fall.

The *Bear* and its crews had many adventures over the ship's long years of Alaska service, but none quite like the rescue of the whalers stranded in the pack ice off Point Barrow in the winter of 1897–1898. A key role in this rescue was played by the same Dr. Call.

In early November 1897 word had reached Washington that eight whaling ships with 265 men had become caught in the ice. The *Bear* had just come back to Seattle from six months in northern waters, but within three weeks it was readied for a return trip to the Bering Sea carrying a volunteer crew. The captain was ordered to reach the highest latitude possible and to drive a herd of reindeer overland to Barrow in the dead of winter to provide food and winter clothing for the whalers.

The *Bear* encountered heavy ice conditions and could only reach Nelson Island, where Surgeon Call and Lieutenants Jarvis and Bertholf were put ashore with seven dogs, two sleds, and essential supplies. Call took along only a small medical bag, assuming that the ships and mission station at Barrow would have the supplies that he would need. The three, together with an Eskimo guide, set off with four sleds for the Yukon River, which they reached at Christmastime. From there it was on to Unalakleet and Cape Nome, where they finally obtained some reindeer near. Call herded 138 reindeer north while Jarvis purchased or otherwise finagled several hundred more from the area around Wales. The officers continued driving the reindeer herd before them in the bitter wind and cold, with their own sleds now being pulled by reindeer. They finally reached Point Barrow on March 29, where they found most of the whalers living ashore. Their mood was surly and quarrelsome, and food was in short supply.

Although exhausted by the journey, Dr. Call immediately undertook a detailed health survey, not only of the whalers but also of the local Eskimos. He also treated many patients with illnesses and injuries during visits to the stranded vessels. Only one death occurred among the whalers after their arrival, and Call performed an autopsy. He also reported at length on the health problems and modes of treatment of the Eskimos, detailing his findings in a report published as a supplement to the official report of Lieutenant Jarvis.

Call, Jarvis, and Bertholf, together with some of the stranded whalers, returned home late that summer on the *Bear*, which had come north again on its annual patrol.[18] President McKinley wrote in a message to Congress, "The year just closed [1898] has been fruitful of noble achievements in the field of war [the Spanish-American War], and while I have commended to your consideration the names of heroes who have shed luster upon the American name in valorous contests and battles by land and sea, it is no less my pleasure to invite your attention to a victory of peace." In response each of the officers received a

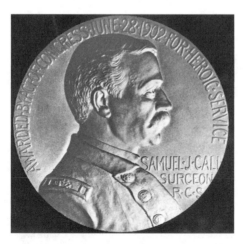

Figure 4. Facsimile of Congressional gold medal struck in honor of Dr. Call. *John W. White and James T. White Collection, University of Alaska Fairbanks*

Congressional Gold Medal struck in his honor "for heroic service" on the expedition to provide relief to the stranded whalers.[19]

Dr. R. N. Hawley, surgeon aboard the *Bear* during its 1899 cruise to the Arctic, gives some idea of the variety of medical experience during a voyage. Overall he considered the health of the crew "remarkably good," with only three serious illnesses and a few minor injuries. The only individual unable to return to duty was the fireman, whom Hawley considered to have malaria resulting from his service in Alabama during the Civil War. In arctic waters many of the crew developed "severe colds and influenza, and a few mild cases of influenza," but all recovered promptly. At Port Clarence, he visited four whaling steamers, where he examined and treated 20 sailors, fitting four of them with trusses for their hernias. He also dressed the knife wounds of a man injured in a fight. At Kotzebue Sound he found 30 cases of scurvy among a group of destitute miners who were taken on board, and by the time the ship reached St. Michael, where he left them with the army doctor, they were showing visible improvement. Whenever the ship stopped long enough at a Native village, Hawley treated all who requested his assistance, including a good number of influenza and pneumonia cases. His report concluded with his concerns about the danger of smallpox being introduced from Puget Sound, where it was then prevalent, to Alaska in the next shipping season, as well as the need to keep the ship's water supply safe from typhoid, which he found to be common in Nome and St. Michael.[20]

Dr. James T. White, the son of a Revenue-Marine captain with years of experience in Alaska, made his first voyage north as an Acting Assistant Surgeon on the *Bear* in 1889, under the command of Captain Healy. White's private diary made during the voyage revealed that the captain was regularly intoxicated and that Lieutenant Cantwell, later to be his commanding officer, was embroiled in a bitter feud with the captain, who was accusing him of

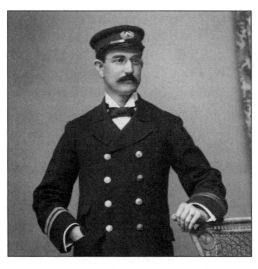

Figure 5. Dr. James T. White, USMHS. *John W. White and James T. White Collection, University of Alaska Fairbanks*

malingering. White and Dr. Call were later asked to carry out a medical examination of Cantwell, and they recommended that he be relieved of duty for "neuralgia," although there was evidence that he also was tippling.[21]

Following some postgraduate training in Philadelphia, Dr. White returned to Alaska in the summer of 1890, this time as surgeon on the cutter *Richard Rush*. The next year he tried to settle down in a private practice in Seattle, but in 1894 he was back with the Marine-Hospital Service and was posted to the *Bear* once again for a few years. He then sailed aboard several commercial ships to the Orient before returning once more to Alaska in 1900, this time as medical officer on the revenue cutter *Nunivak*. That summer he described one of the fiercest epidemics in the history of Alaska, still referred to in Alaska Native oral history as "The Great Sickness." The epidemic, a deadly combination of influenza and measles, spread throughout western and northern parts of the territory, causing the abandonment of many villages. Estimates of deaths ranged up to two thousand, with some areas probably suffering a mortality of 30 to 40 percent.

The *Nunivak*, a rather unattractive, snub-nosed, shallow-draft steamer, was built to navigate the Yukon River. White described his working conditions on the vessel in a small, handwritten note found among his papers. Although the *Nunivak* was supplied with "about every medicine a drug store would want," the dispensary was so cramped it hardly allowed room for one person. A chain divided the available space in half, leaving barely scope for two men to stand upright. There was no place to examine a patient lying down, nor was there a hospital bed for the sick. The dispensary was located at the stern of the vessel, and although a steam heater was available, the heating needs of the rest of the ship left the dispensary so cold that many liquid medications froze and were thus spoiled.[22]

In June and early July of that year, a smallpox scare near Nome had necessitated the establishment of a quarantine station on Egg Island, in Norton Sound (see below), but soon the smallpox situation was dwarfed by an outbreak of influenza followed by measles among the people of the region:

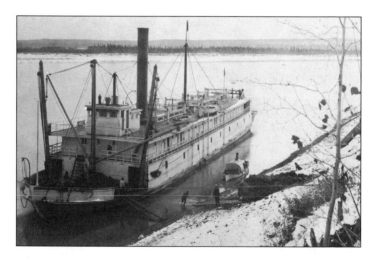

Figure 6. US Revenue Cutter *Nunivak,* designed for use on the Yukon River. *John W. White and James T. White Collection, University of Alaska Fairbanks*

About the middle of July reports were brought in of great destitution, sickness, and death among the natives of the surrounding country. From Surgeon Hawley, of the USS *Bear*, it was learned that this same condition existed along the coast as far north as Cape Prince of Wales and on the Siberian side . . . [O]n St. Lawrence Island the natives were dying so fast, and so many of the remaining were sick, that the dead were left where they lay or simply removed out of doors, out of the way, and there left to the mercies of the dogs.

The diseases spread like a tundra fire through the lower Yukon basin, leaving a staggering mortality, especially in the Alaska Native villages and fish camps:

About 20 miles above Pitka's Point we stopped at a village of 5 houses occupied by 20 people, most of whom were sick with either influenza or measles. In one small house were found 5 or 6 people, some of whom were very sick. The place was dark, damp, and dismal, the fireplace was cold, and an odor of rotting fish permeated everything. The inmates were lying about on their beds, some covered, some uncovered. In one corner was a girl of about fourteen years, entirely nude, whose body was covered with the red rash of measles. Food and medicines were left for the use of these poor people, and we hurried on.[23]

White served a further three years in Alaska on the cutters *Bear* and *McCulloch*, but in 1905 the Revenue-Cutter Service decided they would no longer appoint Acting Assistant Surgeons to its vessels. White, then 38, was too old to apply for a regular Public Health and Marine-Hospital Service commission and returned to California, where he married a doctor and went into private practice. He died there of typhoid fever in 1912.[24]

By 1903, Governor Brady considered the work of the medical officers on the cutters so important that he mentioned it in his *Annual Report*:

These vessels do an immense amount of service and as they travel to many places where there are no doctors or medicine, the surgeons aboard are always appealed to for help, and many of the cases are pitiable. It should be a standing rule with the Treasury Department [which then supervised both the Revenue-Cutter Service and the Marine-Hospital Service] that all doctors aboard these vessels should be expected to give their services to all suffering ones, and especially the natives, without expectation of compensation. Each doctor should be provided with proper vaccine virus [against smallpox], and it should be made known that they are always ready to vaccinate all who have never had the treatment.[25]

Another cutter surgeon of this period who left a personal record of his voyage was Dr. Friench Simpson, who joined the Public Health and Marine-Hospital Service in 1906 and was posted to Alaskan waters on the Cutter *Commodore Perry* during the summer of 1909. One of his adventures that summer was treating a case of ruptured appendicitis in a member of the crew while the ship was in the neighborhood of the Pribilof Islands. After consultation with medical officers on the *Bear* and the *Rush*, Simpson decided that immediate surgery was necessary. Since his ship had "nothing even resembling a sick-bay," he asked the captain to anchor in the lee of St. George Island, and he and Dr. Lanza of the *Rush* set about preparations for surgery. They sterilized their instruments in the galley and then converted the dining room table in the cabin to an operating table. With the Second Engineer giving the anesthetic, the two doctors plunged in and found severe general peritonitis. Although they flushed and drained the peritoneal cavity, within a few hours the patient was nearly moribund from shock. The ship made all steam for Unalaska, where on arrival Simpson and another PHS ship's surgeon performed a colostomy ashore. The patient ultimately made a remarkable recovery.[26]

Assistant Surgeon H. E. Hasseltine was posted as medical officer on the venerable *Rush* from April 1910 through March 1911 and later published an account of his voyage. Hasseltine wrote of disease patterns, general sanitation, housing, clothing, diet, and occupation of the Alaska Natives from Metlakatla to Bristol Bay. He was the first to report poliomyelitis from Alaska, with the earliest cases going back as far as 1908. He also noted the high prevalence of syphilis, tuberculosis, measles, and trachoma among the people, and commented on the threat of spread to the non-Native settlers.[27]

Dr. J. A. Watkins served as medical officer on the 1913 cruise of the *Bear* to the northern Alaskan Coast and islands of the Bering Sea and later reported on the many sick individuals he had treated. He attributed much of the disease he found among the Eskimos to the adverse effects of their contact with miners, whalers, and traders, and "those that follow in the wake of such adventurers." Like others before him he commented on the general sanitation, housing, clothing, and diet of the people he met in the 14 villages he visited. Among the illnesses he encountered, eye inflammation was the most common, followed by pulmonary tuberculosis, bronchitis, and impetigo.[28] During most of the voyage he had the medical companionship of another PHS medical officer, Dr. Emil Krulish. At each Native community they visited, both physicians went ashore to treat the ill, investigate sanitary conditions, and note any infractions of sanitary regulations in the villages. At Point Hope they amputated the leg of an Eskimo man, who on the ship's return south was found to be getting around quite well. The ship's carpenter fashioned a wooden leg for him and it was hoped that he would soon be able to fend for himself. While the *Bear* was caught between the pack ice and the shore east of Point Barrow, some Eskimos arrived in a boat to say that there was much sickness in the village. Dr. Watkins volunteered to accompany them back to the village with an emergency kit. The group reached shore with considerable difficulty and danger, and Captain J. G. Ballinger commended him most highly to the PHS "for his zeal and attention to duty."[29]

In November 1913 an epidemic of measles occurred among the Natives of Kodiak Island, Afognak Island, and Cook Inlet. At the request of the Governor and the Bureau of Education, the Treasury Department dispatched the cutter *Tahoma* from Seattle, carrying on board PHS Passed Assistant Surgeon L. W. Jenkins together with Red Cross food and medical supplies for the stricken communities. When the ship reached Kodiak, Jenkins was joined by Dr. Silverman, a local physician, and Dr. H. O. Schaleben, the district superintendent of schools and physician for the Bureau of Education. By the time the ship arrived, however, the measles epidemic was largely over and the physicians spent their time distributing relief supplies and fumigating all infected houses. Measles had apparently been brought to the area by the steamship *Dora*, proceeding from Seward to Nushugak, which carried the child of a schoolteacher diagnosed with the disease.[30]

Assistant Surgeon T. C. Galloway Jr., after serving as medical officer on the cutter *Unalga* during its Alaskan cruise of 1914, wrote an account of the health of the Aleuts. He noted the severe population decline resulting from repeated epidemics of smallpox, measles, and syphilis in the region over the past century. Galloway found that a "large majority of the chests" that he examined had active signs of tuberculosis and residents of the villages stated that nearly every Native had a chronic cough. He also described the adverse health effects of the foggy, damp, and windy climate, and the semi-subterranean houses that he called "half cave, sod covered, usually damp, dark, and airless." He felt, moreover, that their restricted diet contributed to poor health, since "they are fatalistic and improvident, and live in alternate surfeit and famine." Galloway was realistic in his assessment of the "negligible" value of the treatment and instruction that PHS officers on the revenue cutters could give during their short visits that occurred only once or twice a year, especially since "the natives have to be treated almost against their will."[31]

The 1916 summer cruise of the cutter *Unalga* carried PHS Assistant Surgeon W. F. Fox as medical officer. The ship first visited Kodiak Island, the Aleutians, and the Pribilofs, and Fox commented on disease prevalence, sanitation, water supplies, and the hygienic practices of the people in these areas. At Unalaska he left bottles of silver nitrate solution, together with written instructions on the use of the Credé method for preventing ophthalmia neonatorum, with the priest, marshal, and local midwives. Among his more interesting medical observations were that many local residents suffered from tapeworms, and that diarrhea was widespread from eating an excess of fish and raw turnips, the latter a local favorite. Dental health was especially poor, and Fox recommended that a government dentist make at least an annual visit to the village.[32] On the return voyage the vessel called at Anchorage, at that time a small local supply depot for the Alaska Railroad then under construction.[33]

Another heroic effort in the face of a major epidemic occurred during the great Spanish flu epidemic of 1918 and 1919. The second epidemic wave struck with the arrival of the first ships of the season to the Aleutians and Bristol Bay, with Unalaska being especially hard hit. All Alaska Natives

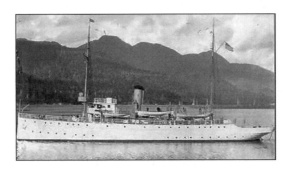

Figure 7. US Coast Guard Cutter *Unalga. USCG photo*

were sick, as well as teachers, government workers and their families, and the local government physician. From May 27 to June 2, 1919, the entire crew of the cutter *Unalga* went ashore with face masks to feed the starving, clean and fumigate homes, cook for the sick, do their laundry, nurse the dying, build coffins, and bury the dead. Captain F. G. Dodge, who himself contracted influenza, wrote in his final report on the mission that he felt certain that without the aid rendered by the doctor and other personnel of the *Unalga*, "there would have been very few left alive at Unalaska and Dutch Harbor."[34] Following the work at Unalaska, the *Unalga* next proceeded to Dillingham, on Bristol Bay. There they found 300 individuals sick, 100 orphans, and many bodies left to be eaten by the dogs. Dodge again sent a detail ashore to bury the dead, shoot dogs, and care for the sick. At least one sailor had to be sent back to the cutter because "his constitution could not stand the work."[35]

The *Bear* was stationed farther north during the epidemic. When the ship called at Port Clarence, Kotzebue, Diomede Island, St. Lawrence Island, Wales, and Point Hope, the surgeon was sent ashore first to assess the situation. The landing party was often greeted by silence and death, with the living lying prostrate in their tents and the dead bodies being eaten by starving dogs.[36]

The physicians working on ships of the Revenue-Cutter Service (which became the Coast Guard in 1916) provided emergency medical care on many other occasions and have engaged in countless search and rescue operations over the years. They were also one of the few dependable sources of medical and, more recently, dental care to the many Alaska Natives who live in the remote coastal villages and islands. Some Revenue-Cutter Service physicians were also engaged in epidemic control, the conduct of important health surveys, and other unusual duties. In one notable example, Surgeon Henry Horne of the cutter *Rush* was ordered by his skipper to enumerate the people of the islands west of Unalaska for the 1900 Federal Census and had the honor of making the first report to the census office at Washington.[37]

Since 1920 a dental officer has accompanied most of the ships of the Bering Sea Patrol, providing dental care to the crew, commercial fishermen, and coastal Alaska Natives.[38] In 1927, when the venerable *Bear* was finally retired from the Bering Sea Patrol, other cutters, notably the *Northland* (the last cutter rigged for sail), took up its duties. The *Northland* had a modern sick bay and dental clinic and after 1929 regularly carried a PHS medical officer and a dental officer.[39] By 1932 Coast Guard cutters were still providing virtually the only medical and dental care to the Alaska Natives of the remote coastal villages. Moreover, these newer ships were better prepared for medical emergencies and some were even equipped with a modern operating room. The Coast Guard was also using aircraft for search and rescue operations and, when appropriate, they brought a physician or nurse to the scene.[40]

In addition to staffing the ships of the Bering Sea Patrol, the PHS assigned a full-time medical officer to the cutter *Haida*, based at Cordova, Alaska. In March 1935 this ship made a special cruise to the Shumagin and Sanak Islands to investigate and render assistance in a reported infantile paralysis epidemic.[41]

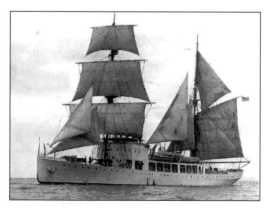

Figure 8. US Coast Guard Cutter *Northland*. *USCG photo*

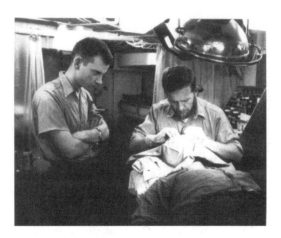

Figure 9. Dr. David Herr performing surgery on board the USCGC *Eastwind. PHS photo*

The Bering Sea Patrol was suspended during World War II, when the cutters were given military assignments in Alaska and elsewhere. Operations resumed after the war, but the changing demands on the Coast Guard and the increasing availability of air transportation finally led to the end of the Bering Sea Patrol in September 1964. As late as 1960, the Bering Sea Patrol cutter carried both a physician and dentist, and that year visited some 25 coastal villages where both PHS officers held clinics ashore.[42] Cutters have continued their many functions in Alaskan waters, especially in interdiction, fisheries patrol, and search and rescue, but the traditional support functions to isolated Alaska Native communities has largely ceased. In 1964 a PHS medical officer was stationed at the Coast Guard station at Annette Island and divided his time between caring for the coastguardsmen there and the Tsimshian Indians at the nearby village of Metlakatla.[43]

PHS physicians still serve aboard the cutters of what is now called the "Alaska Patrol," but they have little interaction with the people of Alaska.[44] It was ironic, however, that as late as the 1960s at least one hard-pressed medical officer from the Alaska Native Health Service was being

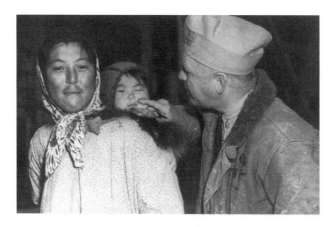

Figure 10. PHS dentist with Eskimo mother and child. *PHS photo*

taken annually away from his duties for six to nine months
to serve, often in utter boredom, aboard cutters on weather
patrol in the North Pacific, particularly at Ocean Station
Victor, until these patrols were discontinued in 1974.

Life on board the cutters was never easy for the physicians. Their quarters were cramped and uncomfortable, the
food was monotonous, and the clinic space was often tiny
and poorly equipped. They were called upon to care for
severe medical or surgical cases far beyond the level of their
training or experience. When the ship was not battling arctic
storms at sea, the doctor was taken ashore in an open boat
to hold long, frustrating clinics in the Alaska Native villages, working among people of another culture and who
had no knowledge of English. Nor should we forget that at
least one PHS Medical Officer died on duty with the
Revenue-Cutter Service in Alaska. On October 10, 1914, Assistant Surgeon L. H. Jenkins (formerly of the *Tahoma*) and
four crew members of the cutter *Manning* drowned when
their small boat swamped in heavy surf off Sarichef, Unimak
Island, in the Aleutians. Two other physicians were rescued
from shipwrecks, including from the *Commodore Perry*, lost
in 1910 off St. Paul Island, and from the *Tahoma*, sunk in the
Aleutians in 1914.[45]

Chapter 3
Marine Hospital Services

As described in the previous chapter, one of the main responsibilities of the physicians on board the cutters was the care of sick or injured seamen on ships in the seas around Alaska. Each year, from approximately May until October, numerous commercial vessels plied the waters of the Gulf of Alaska, the Bering Sea, and, for a shorter season, the Arctic Ocean, in search of fish and sea mammals. In addition, the constant traffic of ships carried passengers and freight to and from Alaska. All of these mariners were eligible under US law for basic medical care by the Marine-Hospital Service for sickness and injuries. Although the medical officers of the cutters were able to provide episodic emergency care and transport, it was clear that expanded services needed to be made available on land.

The earliest mention of a possible marine hospital in Alaska occurred in 1869, just two years after the transfer of the territory to the United States. Noting that the nearest established marine hospital was at Port Townsend, Washington, Dr. Thomas T. Minor of the cutter *Wayanda* saw no current need for an additional one in Alaska, since the volume of commerce was small. Besides, any sailors needing hospital care could be treated at the old Russian hospital in Sitka, now operated by the US Army, at a cost of $1.50 per day.

Following the cruise of the *Rush* in 1879, Captain George W. Bailey, probably prompted by Dr. White, noted in his official account of the voyage that the people of Unalaska, a major stopping point for ships en route to the Bering Sea, were so eager for a hospital that they had started a fund, already at $1,500, to erect a hospital. Bailey wrote, "It would, no doubt, be a worthy charity on the part of the Government to have a surgeon stationed here, say one from the Marine-Hospital Service, who, besides giving his attention to the people, could also attend the sick seamen of the different vessels calling here during the summer, and who are by law entitled to hospital relief."[1] Nothing seems to have come from the suggestion for two more decades.

In 1880 a private physician was designated the MHS representative at Sitka, but no medical activity was reported for that year, except for the collection of $209.58 in taxes.[2] Two years later a medical officer of the Marine-Hospital Service was assigned to Sitka. He remained until June 1883 and in that year treated 48 seamen. In the next fiscal year a private physician was appointed Acting Assistant Surgeon and took over the care of merchant seamen sent to him by the local Collector of Customs.[3] In 1886, Dr. Zina Pitcher described himself as "Acting Assistant Surgeon, USMHS," in a publication describing his medical work with the local Tlingit Indians.[4] By 1888 the local MHS representative was Dr. William Millmore, whose contract called for a reimbursement of $2.50 per day for nursing, quarters, and subsistence for inpatients. That year he had three inpatients, two of whom died, with a combined total of 106 hospital days and 35 office visits.[5]

The workload at Sitka continued to decrease over the next few years. In 1896 an Acting Assistant Surgeon was appointed in Juneau, which had recently replaced Sitka as the territorial capital. St. Ann's hospital was to provide all inpatient services for the princely sum of $2.00 per day, and a local undertaker would be paid $27.50 to care for the remains of any who died. In the first year the doctor treated 28 patients in his office and hospitalized another 15.[6]

In February 1900 the Marine-Hospital Service appointed Dr. Samuel C. Leonhardt as the Acting Assistant Surgeon for the care of cuttermen and merchant seamen at St. Ann's Hospital in Juneau. During the six months ending August 31, 1900, he reported caring for 22 inpatients (one of whom died) for 143 hospital days, plus 51 outpatients. Under the terms of his contract, any patient needing care for more than 30 days would be transferred to the Marine Hospital at Port Townsend.[7]

The commanding officer of the Revenue Cutter *Rush* had reported to the Secretary of the Treasury in the fall of 1892 that there was a pressing need for a "suitable house" at Dutch Harbor or Unalaska where seamen too sick or disabled by injury to be cared for on board ship could be temporarily quartered. He pointed out that during the 1892 navigation season about 50 vessels of the American merchant and whaling fleet had visited the harbor. "The number of persons employed on these vessels will not fall much short of 1,500 persons. They are entitled to medicines and medical treatment, if necessary, and, for this reason, it seems to me a summer hospital ought to be located at Unalaska or Dutch Harbor as the most important and most frequented port in Alaska."[8]

Five years later the Marine-Hospital Service established such a hospital at Dutch Harbor in a house owned by the North American Commercial Company. For the 1897 navigational season, Dr. Gardiner P. Pond was assigned to the facility as "Fleet Surgeon" to treat not only the cuttermen and merchant crews stopping there, but also the local Aleuts. The hospital officially opened on June 26, and over the subsequent 11 weeks or so Pond treated 49 cuttermen, about the same number of merchant seamen, and 27 Alaska Natives. Five cuttermen and four seamen were admitted, one sailor staying for nearly seven weeks with inflammatory rheumatism. When Dr. Pond closed the hospital on September 17, he left his supplies of drugs and instruments in the North American Commercial Company warehouse to be disposed of as the fleet commander ordered.

In forwarding Pond's report to the Secretary of the Treasury, Captain Calvin L. Hooper, commander of the Bering Sea Patrol Fleet, complained that after two years' trial the present system had remained a makeshift operation "unworthy of the Government" and recommended that a marine hospital with a full-time doctor be established at Unalaska. At that time the community included about 375 people, mostly Aleuts. Many ships, including sealers and whalers, stopped there during the summer months en route to the Bering Sea, and some remained in the vicinity all year. Since the daily demands on the doctor came largely from the government school, the Russian Orthodox Church school, and the mission home at Unalaska, a hospital located at Unalaska would serve the cuttermen just as well as the existing one at nearby Dutch Harbor.[9]

This advice was not taken and in the summer of 1900 a new Class 1 hospital opened at Dutch Harbor under the direction of MHS Assistant Surgeon Dunlop Moore. Earlier that fiscal year the Surgeon General had concluded an agreement with the North American Commercial Company for the lease of a large, single-story frame building. When configured as a hospital it had a 20-bed capacity with a medical ward, surgical ward, operating room, dispensary, office, kitchen, two bathrooms, and quarters for stewards and attendants.[10] Dr. Moore arrived on July 16, 1900, at which time he found the hospital building "almost ready for occupancy and of a character suitable for the purposes intended," but since supplies were not expected before August 1, he had to delay the official opening.[11] His staff included another commissioned officer, one steward, and two attendants. Some 26 outpatients were treated in late July and the first inpatient was admitted on August 20.[12] Governor Brady was very pleased with the new facility, "for the number of sailors who pass that way is large and they will feel better to know that there is such a place ever ready for their care and treatment should they become sick or hurt."[13]

The following year Assistant Surgeon Charles N. Vogel reported the Unalaska Hospital workload statistics for FY1901, 1902, and the beginning of 1903. The first year he had treated 11 inpatients and 53 outpatients and during the second year 12 inpatients and 62 outpatients. From July 1 through August 19, 1902, he admitted one patient and treated 17 in the clinic. Besides his hospital work he also served, as did his predecessors, as quarantine officer for the region.[14] The hospital closed in June 1903 because the workload failed to justify its continued operation. That same year, however, a Relief Station was established at Nome, making use of two buildings on the grounds of the old military reservation and the medical equipment from Dutch Harbor.[15] The Nome Relief Station lasted only until September 30, 1904, and the services of the Acting Assistant Surgeon were terminated the following May in favor of a contract with the local mission hospital. That year Ketchikan was added to the list of Alaskan ports where contract services were available.[16]

The Unalaska hospital was apparently the last serious attempt to operate a marine hospital in Alaska. In October 1905 Dr. Joseph H. Romig wrote to Governor Brady asking that the government establish a hospital in the Bristol Bay region, with him as its physician, to care for the many salmon fishermen, prospectors, and settlers who were living there. Romig had come to Bethel in 1896 as the first missionary physician in western Alaska, but in 1905 he was practicing medicine in San Francisco. Like many displaced Alaskans, he was itching to return to Alaska, a goal he ultimately accomplished as a federal school official and later as physician for the Alaska Railroad. Governor Brady endorsed Romig's idea and suggested that the Public Health and Marine-Hospital Service maintain such a hospital, "since the service required at Bristol Bay is so near like caring for sick and disabled sailors that the Marine-Hospital Service is the proper channel through which Congress can provide for these thousands so miserably situated."[17] Officials of the Public Health and Marine-Hospital Service apparently disagreed with the governor's thinking and nothing came of the plan for a marine hospital, although ultimately the Bureau of Education contracted for services there on behalf of the Alaska Natives.[18]

The idea for a marine hospital, however, continued to surface. As late as November 12, 1909, Captain A. J. Henderson, then commanding the cutter *Thetis* on its arctic cruise, recommended that a hospital be established for sailors of the Revenue-Cutter Service, pointing out that hospital furniture stored at Nome could be used in supplying any new facility.[19]

In FY1907 a commissioned officer was assigned to St. Michael, making it a Second Class Relief Station, and a Third Class Station was established at Valdez the same year under the direction of an Acting Assistant Surgeon.[20] Unalaska was added in FY1914, Cordova and Seward in FY1918, Wrangell in FY1921, Petersburg in FY1922, Sitka in FY1923 (reestablished after a lapse of several years), and Kodiak in FY1925. All but the last three of these Relief Stations were under the charge of an Acting Assistant Surgeon, and a Deputy Collector of Customs headed those without a medical officer.[21] The following year Nome was added to the list again and Kodiak was dropped, but in FY1928 Kodiak reappeared, presumably because a new (or at least a willing) physician was found to work under contract.

That year the nine stations were classified as either "Third Class" or "Fourth Class" on the basis of whether a physician was available. Those listed as eligible beneficiaries were seamen from documented American merchant ships and from vessels operated by the Coast and Geodetic Survey, Lighthouse Service, Bureau of Fisheries, and Army. Personnel of the Coast Guard, lighthouse keepers, and injured federal employees under the Federal Employees

Compensation Commission were also beneficiaries. In addition, commissioned and enlisted personnel of the Army, Navy, Marine Corps, and Veterans Bureau were admitted as pay patients upon authorized request. During the summer of 1928, the PHS stationed a dentist at Unalaska for the benefit of merchant seamen.[22]

During FY1930 the station at Kodiak was closed, but with the availability of a new physician the older station at Seward was reactivated. On March 30, 1936, a new law passed by Congress expanded the list of those eligible for care to include crew members of all government vessels other than the navy or those situated in the Panama Canal, and cadets and crews of merchant marine training ships. That year 4,108 days of hospital relief, 7,504 outpatient treatments, and 1,467 physical examinations were provided to beneficiaries in Alaska contract hospitals.[23]

In FY1936 a medical officer and dental officer were assigned to duty ashore at the Coast Guard Dispensary, Unalaska, Alaska, in order to render relief to beneficiaries from the small craft operating out of that port. The medical officer held sick call at the new Indian Affairs Hospital at Unalaska, a considerable improvement compared to the

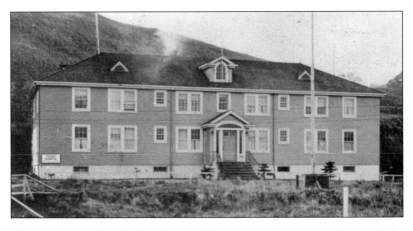

Figure 11. Alaska Native Service Hospital at Unalaska, also used for marine hospital beneficiaries. *Anchorage Museum of History & Art*

service rendered in previous years in the Coast Guard dispensary on the dock.[24] This service continued through FY1939. The hospital, incidentally, was destroyed in the Japanese attack on Dutch Harbor on June 4, 1942. Two years later, four of the stations—Juneau, Ketchikan, Petersburg, and Wrangell—contracted with local dentists on a fee-based arrangement.[25]

The PHS continued to provide contract services for its beneficiaries throughout the war and postwar years right up until the Marine Hospital program was abolished in 1981. It is interesting to note that in 1951 the Territory of Alaska established its own supplementary program, called the Fisherman's Fund, to provide treatment and care for licensed Alaskan commercial fishermen injured while fishing onshore or offshore in Alaska. This program continues to be financed from revenue received from each resident and nonresident commercial fisherman's license and permit fee.

Chapter 4
Quarantine, Disease Control, and General Public Health Support

On June 28, 1900, during the height of the Gold Rush, Lieutenant D. H. Jarvis of the Revenue-Cutter Service reported to the Secretary of the Treasury that the steamer *Ohio*, carrying 700 passengers, had arrived at Nome on June 14 with two well-developed cases of smallpox on board. Jarvis was able to board the ship with the local health officer as she came to anchor, but not before some 15 passengers had escaped into the swarm of boats that surrounded the vessel. Faced with the utter confusion and lack of local government, he considered it his duty to take immediate action to prevent the disease reaching the shore. He selected Egg Island, near St. Michael Harbor and close to the mouth of the Yukon River, as the most desirable place in the region to set up a quarantine station, since it was far enough from shore to preclude the possibility of passengers escaping, had a comparatively safe anchorage, and could almost always be reached from St. Michael. The *Ohio* was ordered to Egg Island and arrived there on June 15. Jarvis, assisted by the commander of the Army contingent at Fort St. Michael, 1st Lieutenant P. M. Cochran, built a camp on the island to which the two smallpox patients were removed. The vessel was then detained in quarantine off the island until it was considered safe for her passengers to land. He engaged Dr. F. N. C. Jeraula, a nurse, and a cook on the island and instituted a proper boarding and inspection service for all arriving vessels. All the passengers of the *Ohio* were then vaccinated, and no new cases occurred.

On June 16 the steamer *Santa Anna*, with 350 passengers and one case of smallpox on board, was placed in quarantine at Egg Island and her smallpox patient removed to the camp on shore. All arriving vessels after that time were found free from disease and their passengers allowed to land. Meanwhile, at Nome, two cases of "varioloid" were found in a cabin at the mouth of the Nome River and were immediately quarantined. These individuals had arrived at Nome on June 13 on the steamer *Oregon*, from Seattle, without any report by the master and before any knowledge of the danger of smallpox had reached authorities. Indeed, the medical officer of the ship had claimed that they were mild cases of chickenpox. No new cases resulted, but Jarvis feared spread of the outbreak, since some 12,000 people were then in Nome and there were proper accommodations for only a quarter of them. In the frenzy for gold the people were in a continual state of unrest and excitement, and if the disease became epidemic, it would most likely spread throughout the region.[1]

In a telegram dated June 29, Jarvis reported ten cases of smallpox and one death within the past three days, all of them passengers from the *Oregon*, which had subsequently sailed for Seattle without them. He urgently requested medical officers and vaccine sufficient for an estimated 15,000 persons. The *Ohio* and *Santa Anna* were released from quarantine after all passengers were vaccinated and the ships "cleaned as well as possible." Three days later he reported a total of twenty cases to date and again requested medical assistance.[2]

In response, on July 11, 1900, Surgeon General Walter Wyman detailed Assistant Surgeon Bayliss Earle from San Francisco as quarantine officer and two weeks later dispatched Assistant Surgeon B. J. Lloyd to assist him. In addition, Assistant Surgeon Carroll Fox was sent to Dutch Harbor as quarantine officer to help Dr. Dunlop Moore, who was already on duty there at the newly established Marine Hospital.

Earle was ordered to take the first available steamer from either San Francisco or Seattle for Cape Nome, confer with Lieutenant Jarvis, and arrange with him and with General Randall for maintaining the maritime quarantine. Before departure he was asked to confer with Dr. Joseph Kinyoun of the Hygienic Laboratory as to the quantity of sulfur and bichloride and the number of Dutch ovens or pots for fumigation that would be needed. Wyman had already sent 1,000 vaccine units to Captain Roberts, of the cutter *Manning* at Nome, and promised to mail an additional 5,000 units if good quality material was not available on the West Coast.[3]

Within a week of the arrival of the *Ohio*, smallpox had appeared in Nome itself. At the time many disappointed prospectors were returning to St. Michael, the gateway to the Yukon River, and officials feared that the disease could spread up the river with disastrous results for the Alaska Natives, especially since influenza and measles were also occurring that summer. On July 2 the army commander of the District of Alaska issued a quarantine order against any ships from Nome or from coastal points westward. Lieutenant Jarvis of the Revenue Cutter *Nunivak* was on the scene and offered to assist in enforcement duties.

The *Nunivak* accordingly took up a position at the mouth of the harbor, and its men, using a steam launch, boarded and inspected every incoming ship. Dr. James T. White initially set the time of quarantine at 14 days, but on July 21 the commanding general arbitrarily reduced the time to eight days, despite White's protest that it was "just long enough to cause considerable inconvenience to commerce and insufficient to prevent the landing of smallpox." Fortunately, the threat from Nome by then was largely past. That quarantine had lasted 24 days, during which time 39 ships were boarded and 29 detained. All of the detained passengers were required to stay aboard their ships, despite vigorous protests, and all mail was fumigated using sulfur dioxide. Only one doubtful case of smallpox appeared, and this proved, ominously, to be measles.[4]

By this time at least 18 cases of smallpox had appeared in Nome and the medical officer there had also begun quarantine inspection of ships that had passed through Dutch Harbor en route north. Smallpox soon after also appeared in Dawson City, in the Yukon Territory, brought there by prospectors entering the Klondike region through Skagway. This situation prompted American authorities to contemplate quarantine inspection of all boats coming down the Yukon River, but they soon realized that every precaution was being taken against spread by the Canadian authorities and the quarantine was dropped.

At Unalaska Dr. Dunlop Moore, who had just arrived to open the Marine Hospital there, proposed to the Surgeon General on July 16 that he begin inspecting vessels at Dutch Harbor. To accomplish this he asked for authorization to hire a rowboat and oarsmen, in the absence of a steam launch.[5]

On July 28, the Secretary of the Treasury issued instructions to Surgeon General Wyman formally establishing quarantine stations at Dutch Harbor and Cape Nome, Alaska. That same day President McKinley authorized the detail of commissioned officers of the MHS to Alaska, since no local health authority existed in the region. Assistant Surgeon Carroll Fox thereupon proceeded from Port Townsend on the Revenue Cutter *McCulloch* to the new Marine Hospital at Dutch Harbor, where Dr. Moore was appointed the quarantine officer in addition to his clinical duties at the hospital. Fox was to assist him until the end of the navigation season, at which time he would return to his home base on a revenue cutter. Assistant Surgeon Lloyd was to sail on to Nome on the *McCulloch* and there help establish a second quarantine station under the direction of Assistant Surgeon Earle, who was already on the site. Each carried 3,000 units of smallpox vaccine.[6]

During the summer cruise of the *Rush* in the Gulf of Alaska and the Panhandle that year, Surgeon Mulroney took the opportunity to vaccinate any Alaska Native who had not previously received it or who had not already had the disease. Some 1,200 individuals were vaccinated "without opposition or reluctance," since many had personal knowledge of the devastation the disease could cause.[7]

A communicable disease, thought by at least some to be smallpox, broke out in December of that year in Saxman, an Alaska Native village near Ketchikan, and affected about 80 persons, a majority of the village. A local physician sent to assist treated and bathed all the patients, fumigated the houses with sulfur dioxide, and took the draconian measure of killing all the dogs in the village. Those who did not contract the disease were vaccinated. A few cases of the disease appeared at Ketchikan, two of which were in the latter stages when Fox arrived. These were isolated in their houses and their houses disinfected.

Around this time an Indian who was to be married left Saxman for Sitka, there developing a form of the disease that he then passed on to many of the Alaska Native inhabitants. Fox examined the man, who had by then entirely recovered, and noted that he was pockmarked, as were a number of others who had had the disease. About 70 cases occurred at Sitka, 24 of whom were isolated on nearby Japonski Island and their houses burned. All the houses in the village were then disinfected whether they had contained smallpox cases or not, and a thorough vaccination campaign proved very successful. Thirty cases were treated in the mission hospital, but others with the disease left to visit friends in other locations.

At Juneau Fox heard of one case in an Indian, who was immediately isolated on Douglas Island and his house thoroughly disinfected. At Douglas City there were eight cases among the Indians, all of whom were isolated on Douglas Island. One sick individual escaped from quarantine and attempted to go to Sumdum, but the local inhabitants would not allow him admittance to their houses. He lay encamped on the beach some distance away and then left for other parts.

At Skagway four cases occurred among Whites, all probably acquired in Seattle or on the steamer. In the large Indian village at Killisnoo, Fox identified some half dozen cases, all mild, and noted that many others had gone into isolation of their own accord some distance from the village.

There were reports of smallpox at Hoonah, Angoon, Cholmondely, and other small Indian settlements, but Fox was unable to obtain transportation to visit them. He tried to obtain passage on the *Rush*, but the captain already had orders to proceed to Valdez to hold court. Fox then suggested that the Marine-Hospital Service charter a vessel with one commissioned officer, an assistant, an interpreter, and twelve attendants to complete the job of inspection, fumigation, and vaccination, but this request was denied. He further recommended that an MHS officer be allowed to remain in Alaska for a time and make a thorough inspection of all Alaska Native villages in November after the Indians' return from their summer's work. His task would be not only to vaccinate those who had been overlooked, but also to discover the first sign of a new outbreak and take immediate action. Fox also noted that the local authorities were disinfecting all Indian curios and furs and at no places would such things be allowed on board a vessel without a certificate showing that they had been disinfected.[8]

In the summer of 1901 two cases of smallpox appeared at Sitka among the crew of the US Fish Commission Steamer *Albatross*, with no indication how the disease had been acquired. After the second case was identified, MHS Acting Assistant Surgeon J. C. Kooshner handed Captain Moser an order that he proceed immediately, flying the yellow flag, to the nearest quarantine station at Port Townsend, Washington. Governor Brady, who had already had smallpox, asked permission to go aboard to speak with the captain before departure, but Kooshner refused. When Brady defied the order, Kooshner bravely quarantined him in an office for 48 hours while his clothes were fumigated.[9]

The disease also spread to Killisnoo, Juneau, and Douglas, where all cases were in Alaska Natives. By June 30, however, Acting Assistant Surgeon Leonhardt could report that the pest house in Juneau was now empty and had been fumigated. In all he had treated 9 cases and kept quarantined for 14 days another 26 Natives who had been exposed to the disease. Leonhardt went on to say that Assistant Surgeon Foster requested him to attach US Marine-Hospital Service stickers to all the articles he disinfected, including some 3,000 furs and curios.[10]

During the 1901 navigation season, 180 vessels at Dutch Harbor and 86 at Cape Nome were inspected and no further evidence of communicable diseases was found.[11] Smallpox, however, did continue to appear sporadically. In December 1901 eight additional cases of smallpox were officially reported from Hoonah.[12] In the same month Dr. Leonhardt reported that a man who was thought to have measles was brought to Juneau from a mining camp. Leonhardt, however, considered him to be suffering from confluent smallpox in the fifth day of eruption. He was placed in a "pest tent" along with three of his companions, pending construction of a pest house. Since the miner had been living in an isolated area for the past month, Leonhardt thought there was little likelihood of spread. Two other cases of smallpox were reported from Skagway that year. The quarantine stations remained active at Dutch Harbor and Cape Nome in FY1902 and inspected 107 vessels.[13]

In April 1911 smallpox threatened Alaska once again. During that spring the disease was prevalent along the West Coast and could easily have been introduced into Alaska, especially with the large numbers of fishermen, miners, and cannery workers who headed north each spring. Public Health and Marine-Hospital Service representatives were directed to notify steamship companies that all crew and passengers be vaccinated or show proof of recent vaccination. US consuls at Vancouver and Victoria were directed to require bills of health for all ships heading for Alaska and that all such vessels stop for inspection at Ketchikan, a community that was becoming the gateway to Alaska. As a result of these measures, 78 vessels were inspected in US ports before departure. The smallpox status of some 7,832 persons was determined, and 5,247 passengers and crew were vaccinated. No cases of smallpox were introduced from the south. These measures were again implemented during the spring of 1912.

Another threat was from the Yukon Territory of Canada. On June 21, 1911, Governor Walter E. Clark of Alaska telegraphed that smallpox was present in Dawson and requested that the Public Health and Marine-Hospital Service furnish assistance in protecting the interior of Alaska. Passed Assistant Surgeon M. H. Foster, already on special duty with the Bureau of Education at Seward, Alaska, was directed by telegraph to sail immediately to Juneau to consult with the governor there, and if necessary proceed to Dawson to investigate conditions. He was further given authority to nominate acting assistant surgeons to enforce the quarantine regulations regarding the introduction of smallpox into the territory of the United States. He appointed two such officials, at Eagle and Skagway, to prevent the introduction of the disease into northern and southeastern Alaska, respectively.

Foster reported that the first case of smallpox reached Dawson April 2, 1911, in a person who was sick at the time of arrival, having come via Seattle before the order requiring vaccination had been issued. His disease was initially diagnosed as la grippe and it was not until several other cases had appeared that the diagnosis of smallpox was established. Action by the Canadian authorities soon controlled the disease in Dawson and no cases were introduced into Alaska.

Sometime after July 1, 1911, however, smallpox was reported at New Rampart House, Yukon Territory, near the international boundary line, but officials of the International Boundary Survey based there, together with Canadian health authorities, were successful in preventing its further spread.[14]

Another communicable disease threatening Alaska around this time was poliomyelitis. This disease was first reported in Sitka in 1908, with five cases and two deaths. Seven cases occurred at Douglas, one at Chichagof, and one at Yakutat (all in Southeast Alaska) in 1910. In the summer of 1912, however, fifteen cases, three of them fatal, occurred in St. Michael and Unalakleet on Norton Sound in western Alaska.[15]

Smallpox appeared in Alaska again in FY1914, with one case reported at the cannery at Uyak Bay, six at the cannery at Hoonah, and two in Juneau. All were in Whites who had entered Alaska as cabin passengers through the port of Seattle. None was vaccinated prior to embarkation, as was usually required of steerage passengers. That year outbreaks of scarlet fever, measles, whooping cough, influenza, mumps, poliomyelitis, and diphtheria were also reported among both Whites and Alaska Natives.

PHS officials gave special attention that year to the inspection of vessels, particularly regulations prohibiting the use of public towels and drinking cups by common carriers engaged in interstate passenger traffic. They also extended advice and assistance to the governor of Alaska, who served *ex officio* as the commissioner of health, in matters regarding quarantine, communicable diseases control, and public health legislation. The Territorial Legislature, in their first session in 1913, had passed an act providing for the registration and restriction of communicable diseases and the registration of vital statistics in Alaska, but the necessary funds for the strict enforcement of these laws were not forthcoming.[16] In FY1916 the commissioner, with the assistance of the PHS, promulgated comprehensive rules that required the reporting of cases of preventable diseases to local health officers and through them to the assistant health commissioners in charge of the health divisions into which the territory was divided.[17]

Alaska, like most of the world, was overwhelmed by the 1918–1919 Spanish flu epidemic. The disease first broke out in October 1918 in the coastal towns of the Gulf of Alaska and in Nome and rapidly spread to some interior settlements. The Bureau of Education medical program was soon overwhelmed, causing Governor Thomas Riggs to call upon the Surgeon General for emergency assistance. The latter authorized the governor to deputize all Alaskan physicians as Temporary Assistant Surgeons at a salary of $100 per month to aid in fighting the epidemic.[18] Sufficient manpower, however, was not available in Alaska, and finally an additional 19 physicians and 3 nurses were secured in Washington State and sent to Alaska on the naval collier *Brutus*. All of the Bureau of Education's physicians, nurses, superintendents, and teachers were then placed at the governor's disposal and rendered exceptional service in fighting the epidemic in the Alaska Native villages. In May 1919 influenza reappeared among the Eskimos in the Bristol Bay region and among the Aleuts at Unalaska. As previously recounted, the revenue cutters *Unalga* and *Bear*, along with several naval vessels, were dispatched to the region carrying physicians and nurses.[19]

In the early months of 1926 smallpox was again widespread along the coast of the Pacific Northwest. In order to forestall a potentially disastrous epidemic in Alaska, territorial health officials requested PHS to cooperate in maintaining quarantine on all ships heading north. During the period from February 18 to June 30, 1926, PHS officials vaccinated 11,851 passengers bound for Alaska, and only three cases appeared in the territory. Within Alaska about 4,000 vaccinations were performed.[20]

In 1925 reports of epidemic influenza were received from the cannery district of Bristol Bay. The governor again sought assistance from the PHS, which requested the Treasury Department to send a revenue cutter to the district. The reports seem to have been overblown, however, and few cases were confirmed.[21]

A famous event in Alaskan history peripherally involved the Public Health Service during FY1925. Surgeon General Hugh S. Cumming reported this incident in a laconic, matter-of-fact manner in his *Annual Report*:

> *Relief Station No. 295, Nome, Alaska.* — Acting Asst. Surg. Curtis Welch in charge. At this port, the most northerly relief station of the Public Health Service, a serious epidemic of diphtheria occurred during the past winter. With the cooperation of the Bureau of Education, the Alaskan Railroad administration, and the Delegate from Alaska, and by assistance from private dog-team drivers along the Yukon River and other Alaskan citizens, a sufficient quantity of antitoxin was secured and delivered in time to control the disease before serious loss of life occurred.[22]

The story, in fact, was more complicated. In the fall of 1924 Dr. Welch, who had lived in Alaska since 1907, examined an Eskimo child with a severe sore throat, but concluded it was not diphtheria, since no siblings were affected. Another child developed similar symptoms in mid-December, and two more in early January, all of whom died. By now Welch was fairly certain he was dealing with diphtheria, but found that the 80,000 units of antitoxin he had on hand were at least six years old, since he had failed to reorder until the previous summer and the serum had not made it onto the fall supply ship. He sent a telegram to Surgeon General Cumming in Washington urgently requesting one million units and also notified the territorial governor in Juneau. Since the only transportation available to Nome during the winter months was mail via dogsled from Nenana, the prospects seemed dim that any antiserum would reach Nome in time to be useful. Welch imposed a strict quarantine on the community and worked to near exhaustion caring for the sick, even administering the out-dated antitoxin, which in fact seemed to help in some cases. In the next few weeks there was a flurry of publicity regarding Nome's plight and the story of the epidemic captivated national attention. All sorts of proposals were made, including bringing a ship as far north as the ice permitted and using aircraft in the dead of winter darkness to fly the serum from Fairbanks. Finally, a supply of 300,000 units of serum was located in Anchorage and transported by the new Alaska Railroad to Nenana, where the precious package was passed from one dog driver to the next all the way to Nome. In total, 20 mushers participated in the 674-mile sprint. The serum finally reached Nome on February 2 and about two weeks later the quarantine was lifted. The total number of cases, according to the governor, was 34, with five deaths. Only a few cases were actually given the new antitoxin, which had arrived after the epidemic was largely over.[23]

Dr. Welch, although lionized by the public, had his shortcomings. Some wondered why he was drawn to Alaska in the first place, since he had a Yale medical degree and excellent prospects for a profitable practice. It also seems likely that after 18 years on the isolated northwest coast of Alaska he was not as up to date as he might have been. He clearly missed the diagnosis on the first few cases and may have been negligent in keeping his antitoxin supplies up to date. He had a microscope but no facilities for bacteriological examination. When the epidemic was over, Surgeon General Cumming suggested in a letter that he might want to upgrade his laboratory facilities, to which Welch replied that it had been a long time since he had done that kind of work and "I hardly feel competent to make cultures." Cumming then offered him an opportunity to become trained in "easily applied laboratory procedures."[24]

Another program of the Public Health Service around this time was the examination and instruction in first aid and ship sanitation for ships' officers and candidates for licenses on American vessels. Among the American ports where this activity was carried out in FY1927 was Juneau, Alaska,[25] where it continued for several years thereafter. As early as 1900 the MHS had become interested in the health of the many Asians brought to Alaska each summer to work in the salmon canneries of the Panhandle, Kodiak Island, and Bristol Bay. In October of that year, Assistant Surgeon L. L. Lumsden reported on this problem. As many as 3,000 Chinese sailed north from San Francisco in March or April 1900. Although bubonic plague was known in the city before departure, no precautions were apparently taken. On their return voyages in September, however, the workers were examined for swollen glands, since a number of workers had died on the return voyage and were buried at sea. No abnormal glands were found, but the quarantine officers noted that as many as five percent of the workers had severe weakness and edema of the lower extremities. Two such patients died while in quarantine, and autopsy revealed excess fluid in the body cavities and an acute myocarditis. Lumsden concluded that malnutrition was the dominant feature, perhaps manifesting itself as beriberi. He deplored the filthy living conditions aboard the ships, but curiously did not even speculate that conditions at the Alaskan canneries themselves might also have contributed to the poor health of the workers.[26]

A few years later Assistant Surgeon Donald H. Currie, based in Washington, D.C., reported the clinical details of nine cases in Chinese cannery workers returning from Alaska. Four of the patients died, although in only one case could an autopsy be performed. None of the cases had any immediate connection with each other, and their ages ranged from 23 to 57. All had edema of the legs and cardiac enlargement, but also sensory and motor abnormalities, including paresthesias, muscle weakness, and areflexia. Significantly, the illness had begun in several cases before the workers had embarked for home. Living conditions both on the ships and at the canneries were very poor, with long hours, severe crowding, and a diet made up primarily of rice, dried Chinese vegetables, salt pork, and bacon. Currie was reasonably certain that the disease was beriberi.[27] Because of concern about the introduction of communicable diseases into Alaska, PHS officials at port cities began examining in the spring of 1926 all nonresident employees engaged in the fisheries in the territory. Practically all companies involved cooperated with this endeavor and that year some 8,909 persons were screened for communicable diseases, and were vaccinated as required. This resulted in improved health in nearly all the districts.[28] In 1927 another 3,905 persons were examined and 3,615 were vaccinated against smallpox. Less than 0.5 percent were rejected for health reasons.[29] By 1936 over 11,000 workers were being examined each year in as many as seven West Coast port cities. This service continued until the outbreak of the war in 1941.

The principal ports of entry for foreigners into Alaska remained Ketchikan and Nome for many years, and in both places the Acting Assistant Surgeon served as quarantine officer. In FY1931, Sitka, Wrangell, Seward, Juneau, and Cordova also became official ports of entry. That same year the increasing use of aircraft in Alaska led to the expansion of quarantine service to communities with a major airport. Skagway Airport and the seaplane base at Wrangell were added the following year.[30] In FY1935 the new airport in Juneau and the airport at Fairbanks were also designated ports of foreign entry, although the PHS would not concur with the choice of Fairbanks until funds for an Acting Assistant Surgeon were forthcoming. In FY1939 the small airport at Fort Yukon was added to the list, but no PHS medical officer was ever stationed there.[31]

In 1930 Congress passed legislation allowing the Department of the Interior to pay, from its appropriation, the salary of a PHS officer detailed to supervise the care and custody of those persons judged legally insane in Alaska, and by 1934 such an individual was on duty in Juneau.[32]

Since no actual mental hospital existed in Alaska at this time, all those needing institutional care were sent to Morningside Hospital, near Portland, Oregon. Although Alaska had had a health authority of some kind since 1913, it was largely ineffective because of lack of appropriations. The passage of the Social Security Act by Congress at last provided a mechanism by which the territory could receive adequate funding for a health department. The law went into effect on February 1, 1936, and Title VI, "Public Health Work," set up a fund to assist states, counties, health districts, and other political subdivisions to establish and maintain adequate public health services, including training of personnel. The Surgeon General determined the amount of such allotments based on population and on the special health problems and financial needs of the region. Title V, "Grants to States for Maternal and Child Welfare," also allowed for grants in the areas of general maternal and child health, crippled children services, and vocational rehabilitation.[33] Alaska's share of the original $8 million appropriated for Title VI was a little over $10,000 in the last five months of FY1936, but increased to $23,592 for FY1937. As early as 1936, medical officers and environmental health officers were assigned to the fledgling department. These funds gradually increased, reaching $41,300 by FY1941, and continued as the principal support for the Territorial Health Department until well after World War II.[34]

In FY1939 Alaska began reporting the incidence of sexually transmitted diseases to the PHS, the result of an increasing emphasis in this area by the federal government occasioned by defense mobilization. Thanks to Title VI and the new federal Venereal Disease Control Act, Alaska now had not only the laboratory facilities necessary to make the diagnosis of syphilis and gonorrhea, but also funds for the purchase of drugs for treatment. That year the territory reported 115 cases of syphilis and 231 cases of gonorrhea.[35]

Chapter 5
World War II and Its Aftermath

Because of the strategic importance of Alaska, the outbreak of war in late 1941 intensified the activities of the Public Health Service in the territory. Indeed, Alaska became a battleground itself when in June 1942 the Japanese bombed Dutch Harbor and occupied the two outermost Aleutian Islands. Health services for Alaska Natives were drastically cut back, since many ANS physicians and nurses enlisted in the armed services and very few replacements were available nationally for recruitment. Nurses carried on the work at several hospitals that had lost their physicians, but they too were in short supply, especially public health nurses, who had long been the foundation of public health work in the territory.

A major PHS activity in the early years of the war was its support of the construction of the Alcan Highway. In April 1942 the Federal Works Agency asked Surgeon General Thomas Parran to assist in developing a health care program for the civilian workers then engaged in constructing the 1500-mile military highway from Dawson Creek, British Columbia, to Delta, Alaska, to connect a string of isolated airfields that were already built. The Army Corps of Engineers assigned the bulk of this thankless task to its African-American engineering regiments under the overall command of White officers.

Much of the route was through virgin forest swarming with mosquitoes, whereas in more open areas the denuded permafrost caused seemingly hopeless quagmires of mud in the warmer months. To accomplish this Herculean task, some 16,000 civilian workers were employed at the peak of construction in the summer of 1943. Most of the basic road had been completed by the end of 1942, and during the following year it was passable for truck convoys. Although the road did not play a large part in the war, it was later upgraded, and as the Alaska Highway it became essential to the state's economic development.

The role of the PHS was to provide hospitals and clinics for the civilian construction workers and to supervise all the sanitation aspects of the project. Under the agreement reached with the Public Roads Administration (PRA) the PHS provided the professional staff, including physicians, dentists, sanitary engineers, and administrative staff, while the PRA built the necessary facilities, recruited nonprofessional staff, and provided transportation. Dr. Edwin H. Carnes, a PHS officer, was named overall director of the health and sanitation program, assisted by chief sanitation officer Robert W. Kehr and assistant medical officer Marion B. Noyes.

Carnes reported for duty on June 1, 1942, several months after the construction season had begun. His task was to set up health facilities to care for thousands of men scattered in more than 100 isolated camps, recruit staff, create supply lines, and obtain the necessary equipment and supplies. After he and his senior staff visited the region by airplane, he made his headquarters in Whitehorse, Yukon Territory. In his plan he proposed building two new 50-bed hospitals, at Fort Nelson and at Whitehorse, as well as making contractual arrangements with existing hospitals at Dawson Creek, Fort St. John, Whitehorse, and Fairbanks. Small dispensaries were to be set up along the route so that no section would be more than 100 miles from a medical care facility. Each construction camp had a first-aid station with a trained attendant, and the larger ones were provided with an ambulance. When the program was fully operational, its clinical staff included 13 medical officers, 3 dental officers, 23 nurses, and 2 administrative assistants. The medical facilities handled much trauma, of course, but also general medical and surgical diseases, and even elective surgery as circumstances permitted.

A sanitary engineer was stationed in each of three major sections of the highway. They made periodic inspections of all the construction camps, reported any deviations from accepted standards, and submitted recommendations for resolving problems. They also provided technical assistance regarding water supplies and sewage disposal issues, as well as submitting plans and designs for improved systems.

These sanitary engineers were required to travel frequently by small aircraft, sometimes under marginal weather conditions. On one of these trips Passed Assistant Sanitary Engineer Robert W. Kehr was killed when the plane on which he was flying crashed with the loss of all on board. Shortly afterward the community of Fort Nelson, British Columbia, named its hospital the Kehr General Hospital.

Although the provision of medical care for the civilian workers of the Public Roads Administration was primarily a function of the PHS, the Army Medical Corps also provided some care to civilian workers who were employed by the Corps of Engineers on various projects in the region, including the highway. To avoid any duplication of effort and to coordinate the activities of the services, the Secretary of War in March 1943 requested that the PHS commissioned officers engaged in the Alcan Highway project be assigned to the Army Corps of Engineers until the project came to a close late in 1943. In November and December the PHS officers were reassigned to duty in the continental United States. Dr. Carnes left for another assignment on December 4 following the transfer of all PHS facilities and equipment to the Army.[1]

The Territory of Alaska was originally included under PHS District #5, based in San Francisco. On October 1, 1943, a new District, #11, was established for the territory with headquarters in Juneau. The principal function of the new district office was to assist the Territorial Department of Health in formulating sound public health programs in accordance with the regulations governing the expenditure of federal funds, particularly those under Titles V and VI. Other priorities included the venereal disease program, coordination of civilian and military health programs, the disbursement of emergency funds, and the assignment of health personnel to the territory. The new district director, Medical Director Edgar W. Norris, also served as medical director of the Office of Indian Affairs in Alaska so that he could coordinate the work of the Territorial Health Department and the Alaska Native Service (BIA) programs. The district staff included three medical officers, three sanitary engineers, and four public health nurses who were all assigned to the Territorial Department of Health. In addition there were six remaining part-time Acting Assistant Surgeons located at Ketchikan, Wrangell, Petersburg, Juneau, Cordova, and Seward.[2]

A prominent member of Norris's staff was Senior Surgeon George A. Hays, who began his career in Alaska in the 1930s as director of Crippled Children's Services for the Territorial Health Department and later became the Executive Officer of the Territorial Department of Health. In 1943 he coauthored, with Carl E. Buck, a comprehensive postwar health plan for Alaska, much of which later was realized.[3] The most pressing health problem was tuberculosis, with an estimate of no less than 2,000 active cases scattered throughout the territory, mostly in the Native population. At that time there were no sanatoria in Alaska and the few hospital beds that were available could accommodate only about 5 percent of the cases needing hospital care.

Although he could be abrasive, Hays had many good ideas and the ability to see them through. In 1944 he was able to secure PHS funds for the acquisition of an army surplus vessel that was converted into the *Hygiene*, the first of several health ships used by the Territorial Health Department in the postwar era. In 1944 he was also instrumental in acquiring the surplus army hospital at Skagway that the Alaska Native Service opened in April 1945 as a tuberculosis sanatorium for Alaska Natives.[4] The activities of the *Hygiene* and the sanatorium at Skagway were, in large part, made possible by the PHS Tuberculosis Control Section in the Bureau of State Services, which, after its establishment on July 1, 1944, authorized tuberculosis grants to states and territories during FY1945. Other sources of funds drawn on by the District Office were those authorized by Section 314 of the Public Health Service Act of 1944 (58 Stat 632).[5]

In FY1946 emergency health and sanitation funds were gradually withdrawn and personnel assigned to emergency activities were gradually released. The district office continued to cooperate in surveys of postwar sanitation needs, surveys of hospital facilities, tuberculosis control, and surplus-property disposal. PHS District #11 was abolished on June 30, 1946, and the remaining functions reverted to District #5, which was based in San Francisco.[6]

In March 1945 the Alaska Territorial Legislature created a permanent Department of Health and Board of Health, which came into existence on July 1 of that year. Governor Ernest Gruening, a physician who had never practiced, selected Dr. C. Earl Albrecht as commissioner. Throughout the last two years of the war Albrecht, then the Post Surgeon at Fort Richardson Army base, conferred regularly with George Hays, Edgar Norris, and other PHS officials in Juneau about the form the health department should take at the end of hostilities. They were instrumental in acquiring surplus military buildings and equipment for the use of the new department.

In 1946 the PHS assigned a young tuberculosis specialist, Assistant Surgeon Leo Gehrig, as the Tuberculosis Control Officer for the territory. Dr. Gehrig planned and organized the hugely successful campaign against tuberculosis in Alaska and in later years went on to a distinguished career as Director of the Office of International Health and Deputy Surgeon General.[7] The PHS continued to invest large sums in Alaska under authority of Section 314. In FY1947 the Alaska Department of Health received $47,835 in general health funds, $24,470 for venereal disease control, and $108,575 for tuberculosis control.[8] During this time the new Alaska Department of Health was operating smoothly under the able leadership of Commissioner Albrecht, who, on his regular fund-raising trips to Washington in the 1940s, always made it a point to visit Surgeon General Parran. In 1949 Governor Gruening specifically asked for the continued cooperation of the PHS in providing grants and field services until Alaska was able to mount a public health program comparable to those of other states.[9]

From April through June 1947, an interagency nutrition survey team, jointly funded by the PHS and the Children's Bureau, determined the general nutritional status of the Eskimos in seven western Alaskan villages. Because of the high incidence of corneal opacities in the population, the survey expanded its scope to include an ophthalmologic survey.[10]

Among the other ways in which the PHS was involved in Alaska in this period was as a co-sponsor, along with the Bureau of Indian Affairs and the Phipps Institute, of a long-term study under the direction of Joseph Aronson of the effectiveness of BCG among the US Indian population, and to assist the territorial authorities in setting up an effective BCG program beyond the research protocol. Senior Surgeon T. H. Rose of the PHS District Office in San Francisco worked closely with Commissioner Albrecht on the Alaska Hill-Burton hospital construction program, with the first grant for Alaska being awarded in FY1949. Continuing a program that began during World War II, the PHS provided funds and penicillin for hospitals and private physicians for the treatment of syphilis.[11]

In 1948, following persistent and effective lobbying led by the commissioner of health, Congress appropriated $1,150,000 to the PHS for what was called "The Alaska Health and Sanitation Activities Program." This grant recognized that many diseases that could be controlled by modern public health methods continued to be major health problems in Alaska. Tuberculosis, especially, still ranked first among the causes of death in Alaska, yet was seventh in the rest of the United States. Increases in military activity in Alaska and the influx of civilians since 1945 added to the difficulties of sanitation and communicable disease control. Further, many other aspects of arctic health continued to be unstudied and unsolved.

This health initiative included cooperation with the Alaska Department of Health and the implementation of a research program to conduct basic and applied studies on arctic health. In 1949 some 21 Public Health Service specialists were assigned to the department to assist in the organization and operation of the program. Grants-in-aid in the amount of $775,000 were allotted to the territory to extend and strengthen public health services. The availability of PHS funds allowed the territory to obtain and equip, through war surplus channels, several mobile health clinics—including three ships, a truck unit, and a special

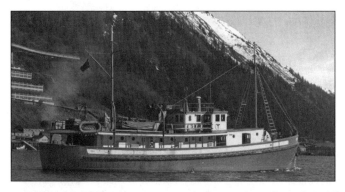

Figure 12. The M/V *Hygiene*, a converted army vessel used as a floating clinic by the Alaska Department of Health. *Alaska Department of Health photo, courtesy of Margery Albrecht*

railway car—to serve isolated communities along the coast and interior railroad lines. A comprehensive BCG vaccination program was also undertaken to combat tuberculosis throughout the territory. (The research elements of the Alaska Program will be discussed in a later chapter.)[12]

The PHS also loaned several officers, including Dr. Florence Marcus, to assist with the BCG program on the M/V *Hygiene* and Dr. Edward T. Blomquist, a tuberculosis consultant from PHS District #5, to help with a wide-ranging tuberculosis survey. In 1947 a consultant record analyst from the PHS spent six months in Juneau helping territorial health officials set up a tuberculosis registry and training clerks.[13]

In 1952 the PHS lent a nurse to the Alaska Department of Health for four months to train public health nurses in the proper techniques for administering BCG. At the same time cuts in PHS funds available from Washington caused the temporary suspension of operation of all three health ships.[14] In May 1954, however, the PHS loaned the health department a state-of-the-art mobile x-ray unit, which over the coming year was used to take over 27,000 chest x-rays to screen not only for tuberculosis, but also for lung cancer and heart disease.[15]

In 1953 and again in 1954, at the request of the Department of the Interior, a team of experts from the University of Pittsburgh Graduate School of Public Health, headed by its dean, former Surgeon General Thomas Parran,[16] visited Alaska to conduct a comprehensive survey of health conditions and programs. Their findings, commonly known as the Parran Report, became an indispensable and wide-ranging plan for the development of modern health services in Alaska, especially in the fight against tuberculosis.[17]

In later years the Alaska Department of Health (and its successor agencies) benefited from a variety of PHS grants, mostly in the area of disease control. A notable example was a special grant from the CDC to fund so-called "Hot-Spot teams," a rapid deployment force consisting of phy-

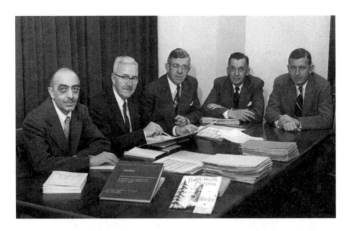

Figure 13. Members of the Parran Survey Committee. L-R: Antonio Ciocco, Former Surgeon General Thomas Parran, Commissioner Earl Albrecht, James A. Crabtree, and Walter J. McNerney. *Alaska Department of Health Photo, courtesy of Margery Albrecht*

sicians, public health nurses, and x-ray technicians, to provide teams to investigate, on short notice, outbreaks of tuberculosis in the Alaska villages. This program was established in 1965 and remained an important part of the state tuberculosis control program for several years. A PHS physician named Keith R. Hooker has left an account of one such investigation.[18]

Following a mental health survey by the Public Health Survey in FY1957, Alaska received authority and a grant of $57,000 to develop an integrated mental health program, including construction of mental health facilities within the territory.[19] In addition, after Alaska became a state in 1959, the PHS made a grant for $1 million for the state's mental health program, followed by a series of annual transitional grants to facilitate an orderly assumption of certain responsibilities in mental health previously carried out by the federal government.[20]

Another area in which the PHS has given notable service is the assignment of CDC Epidemic Intelligence Service (EIS) officers, who have played an invaluable role in investigating disease outbreaks in Alaska. The first of these,

Thomas Bender and T. Stephen Jones, were assigned to the Arctic Health Research Center in 1969. They were followed by Paul Steer in 1971, and then by Richard Brodsky and David Barrett in 1973. Steer later went into private practice in Anchorage, while Brodsky and Barrett had long and notable careers with the Indian Health Service in Alaska. Another member of the class of 1973 was Mickey Eisenberg, the first EIS officer to be assigned to the state Division of Public Health.[21] In 1975 John Middaugh was initially posted to the state as an EIS officer, and after three years on the job and further training returned in 1980 as the state's first full-time epidemiologist. He held that position until 2004, longer than any other state epidemiologist in the nation.[22]

In 1970 the National Health Service Corps was established by Congress as an innovative experiment in the delivery of health care to areas in the United States that were inadequately provided with physicians and other health care professionals. The Washington-Alaska Regional Medical Program office, set up under authority of the Heart Disease, Cancer, and Stroke Amendments of 1965 (PL 89-239), cooperated with the Alaska Division of Public Health and the Alaska Health Manpower Corporation to strengthen rural health care in Alaska, especially through the use of midlevel practitioners. This group requested that an NHSC physician be assigned to Alaska to develop this project, and in August 1972 a PHS officer, Dr. Thomas S. Nighswander, arrived in Anchorage. Over the next three years Nighswander worked with three remote communities— Unalaska, Galena, and Yakutat—to develop a community-based health clinic staffed by a physician's assistant. All of these projects were established on a firm basis and have continued in some form up to the present time. In 1975 Nighswander left the National Health Service Corps and after some further training transferred to the Indian Health Service, where he has had a long and distinguished record at the Alaska Native Medical Center. His NHSC position was filled by Dr. Gerald Bell.

Chapter 6
The PHS and the Bureaus of Education and Indian Affairs

etween 1910 and 1955 a major contribution of the Public Health Service in Alaska was in support of the work of the Alaska Native health programs of the Bureau of Education and the Bureau of Indian Affairs. The health programs operated by these agencies were basically an appendage of the educational system for Alaska Natives. They were chronically underfunded and supervised by officials who, although men of good faith, often had little understanding of health affairs.

As set out previously, the earliest involvement of the PHS with health care for Alaska Natives comes from the reports of medical officers aboard the ships of the Revenue-Cutter Service. During FY1882, when a medical officer was stationed at Sitka, the Department of the Interior asked the Marine-Hospital Service to supply drugs for the use of the Indians, and that the medical officer himself provide care to the local Indians "gratuitously." Since the Interior Department had no appropriations for this purpose, Surgeon General John B. Hamilton refused the request, although he noted, "There is great need of systematic medical relief for these helpless people, as the devastations of syphilis and small-pox among them well attest." He went on to quote at length a communication from Ivan Petroff who, for the most part, had personally conducted the 1880 US Census in Alaska. Petroff pointed out that smallpox vaccination was urgently needed among the Alaska Natives, as "smallpox always exists" among the Chinese sent up from San Francisco each summer to work in the salmon canneries of Kodiak Island. He urged that an MHS medical officer be assigned to western Alaska to vaccinate the local Alaska Natives and render medical care as opportunity presented. He noted further that they could travel at the expense of local trading companies, which freely provided such services to government officials. Nothing seems to have come of the proposal.[1]

When Assistant Surgeon Carroll Fox was detailed to southeastern Alaska in May 1901 to investigate a smallpox outbreak, he was impressed by the severity and extent of tuberculosis in the Native population.[2] Soon after his departure from Alaska, Dr. Fox wrote an article in which he expressed the hope that the Marine-Hospital Service would carry out a scientific study of this "loathsome and contagious disease" among Alaska Natives, which he attributed in large part to the lack of village sanitation, their crowded homes, and their habit of promiscuous spitting. He felt that a government health official stationed on the scene, "clothed with the proper authority," could have a major impact on changing the attitudes of the local population toward hygienic living. He even went so far as to suggest that a tuberculosis hospital be established, though he stopped short of recommending that the Marine-Hospital Service should be responsible for it.[3] Governor Brady had no such scruples and recommended that Congress be asked to appropriate a sufficient sum for a small hospital "to be under the care and control of this branch of the service."[4] This idea arrived stillborn in Washington.

In 1905 the Secretary of the Treasury asked for authority to spend a portion of the Public Health and Marine-Hospital Service (PH & MHS) epidemic fund to prevent the spread of contagious and infectious disease in Alaska, but the request was denied. During the 61st Session of Congress (1909–1911), as a result of consultations among the Departments of the Interior, Justice, and Treasury, it was determined that none of these agencies had either the authority or the appropriations to care adequately for the health of Alaska Natives. Consequently, an appropriations amendment was submitted asking for $50,000 "for medical and surgical relief and sanitary measures relating to the Eskimos, Aleuts, Indians, and other natives of Alaska; for the care of lepers in Alaska; and to prevent the spread of contagious or infectious disease from one part of Alaska to another," all under the supervision of the Public Health and Marine-Hospital Service. This proposal was later modified to place the appropriations under the Commissioner of Education, but none of the measures passed.[5]

In the summer of 1909 the PH & MHS had received an urgent appeal from the governor, the superintendent of education for southwestern Alaska, and from the people of Seward that federal officials take adequate measures regarding certain persons in the Cook Inlet region suspected of having leprosy. Nothing could be done at that time, but as a result of this reopening of the question of the prevalence of preventable disease, the Secretary of the Interior requested, in March 1911, that a medical officer of the service be detailed to work under the direction of the Commissioner of Education. This individual was to supervise all medical, surgical, and sanitary measures relating to the Natives of southern Alaska, study the distribution of disease in Alaska and the conditions favoring its spread, and initiate adequate measures for its prevention. Passed Assistant Surgeon Milton H. Foster was chosen to fill this position.[6]

He was immediately posted to Seward whence, during the summer of 1911, he traveled mainly by ship to some 27 communities throughout southern Alaska. In his report, submitted at the end of August, he made detailed observations on local housing, clothing, food, occupations, water supply, waste disposal, general sanitation, and personal hygiene. He also made note of the prevalent diseases, with special emphasis on tuberculosis, syphilis, and trachoma.

He estimated that the mortality among Alaska Natives was over 80 per 1000, principally from tuberculosis. As a result of his investigations, he recommended that a tuberculosis sanatorium and a home for "destitute and crippled" Natives be built, and that medical services should be expanded. One of his more controversial ideas was that traveling physicians should no longer make periodic brief visits to villages because he felt that the practice was expensive and medically nonproductive; instead, he recommended that nurses remain in villages for up to three months at a time to care for chronic diseases and provide health education. He also endorsed and urged expansion of the practice that each school set aside a room as a dispensary supplied with a simple medicine chest and medical handbook for use by the teachers.

In some ways his most important recommendation was that Congress authorize the Surgeon General to assign a commissioned officer as commissioner of health for the District of Alaska with wide-ranging responsibilities and authority in disease control. Interestingly, he suggested that such an individual receive a 50 percent increase over his regular pay.[7] In a separate report he provided a detailed account of two cases of possible leprosy reported near Cook Inlet. After a careful clinical examination of both individuals, he concluded that one had syphilis and that the other had vitiligo with ataxia.[8]

As a direct result of Foster's report, newly appointed Surgeon General Rupert Blue detailed Passed Assistant Surgeon Emil Krulish in March 1912 to an extended assignment in Alaska as health director for the Bureau of Education. Krulish, then 34 years old, was a seven-year veteran of the Public Health and Marine-Hospital Service. His new responsibilities were daunting, since he was to supervise all quarantine stations in Alaska, manage epidemic outbreaks of disease, and enforce federal regulations to prevent the spread of contagious diseases to and from Alaska, as well as within Alaska. In addition, he was to supervise all measures relating to the medical and surgical relief of the Alaska Natives, conduct studies of the prevalence of disease among Natives, instruct school teachers of the Alaska School Service in first aid to the injured and sick, advise the Superintendent of Education in the territory in all matters pertaining to hygiene, sanitation, maintenance of hospitals, and "other matters of like character."[9]

In 1913, less than a year after his arrival in Alaska, Krulish teamed up with Daniel Neuman, a Bureau of Education physician in Nome, to publish a 179-page *Medical Handbook* designed to assist teachers in the practical recognition and care of common medical problems. This small book is filled with practical advice on both preventing and treating the diseases current among the Alaska Natives. A particularly interesting section was called "Hints on doctoring," which includes the admonition "Begin all treatments with a thorough cleansing of the bowel."[10] The teachers gave the booklet rave reviews over the next few years.

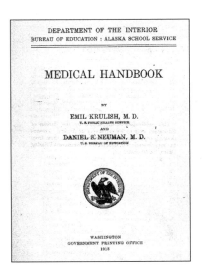

Figure 14. *Medical Handbook* for teachers, by Emil Krulish and Daniel S. Neuman. *Author's collection*

In a series of reports during the course of his initial three-year assignment, Krulish presented the findings of his extensive surveys of sanitation and health problems in Native Alaskans. He covered a wide area, extending from Southeast Alaska to Barrow, traveling by revenue cutter, small boat, and dog team. His accounts, based as they are on direct observation of village conditions and on the diagnosis and treatment of many individual patients, are detailed and vivid. Some of these articles that were presented in national publications, such as *Public Health Reports*,[11] ultimately found their way to Congress and were instrumental, in 1915, in obtaining the first health-specific funding for the Bureau of Education in Alaska.

On his visits to the villages, Krulish would first inspect the sanitary conditions and then visit all the bed-ridden in their homes. Next, he would set up a clinic in the school classroom and examine all the children, with particular attention to the heart, lungs, teeth, tonsils, and eyes, including vision tests. Krulish performed needed surgery on a rough schoolroom table covered with blankets, using a pocket flashlight for illumination. Usually the surgery was restricted to tonsillectomy and adenoidectomy, but on one occasion he amputated the leg of a boy for tuberculosis of the ankle. During the evenings he would give talks to the parents on hygiene, with particular emphasis on tuberculosis, using teaching materials he had specially adapted to use with the Eskimos.[12]

With consultation from Dr. Krulish, PHS officials continued to work with the Bureau of Education in Washington to develop plans and budgets for improving medical services for Alaska Natives. At the request of the Commissioner of Education, they presented and defended these plans at hearings before the Committee on Appropriations in Congress.[13] These efforts led in FY1915 to the first appropriation of $25,000 for health and "medical relief" in Alaska, a sum far below the estimate of need. Bureau of

Education and PHS officials then met to consider how best
to use these funds and decided to build and equip a hospital at Juneau to serve the estimated 5,000 Alaska Natives
living in Southeast Alaska.[14]

Krulish prepared the overall health budget estimates
annually for submission to Congress. He drafted plans for
the proposed hospital to be erected at Juneau and even
selected its furniture, fixtures, and equipment. The hospital, completed in 1916, was a two-story frame structure with
one story devoted to the care of patients and the other to
living quarters for the staff and attendants. Following its
completion Krulish returned to Juneau at the request of the
commissioner to make an inspection of the hospital and
assist in its organization. It opened to receive patients in
May.[15]

In FY1916 Dr. Krulish was transferred from Juneau to
Seattle so that he could be in more direct communication
with officials of the Bureau of Education in charge of the
Alaska School Service, who were stationed in Seattle. He
continued to work closely with school officials on matters
pertaining to hygiene, sanitation, maintenance of hospitals,
and the general administration of the medical service in

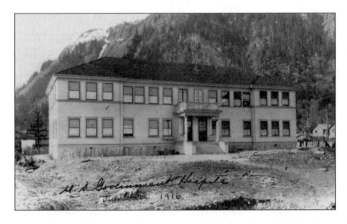

Figure 15. The Bureau of Education Hospital in Juneau, built in 1916,
as the first new government hospital for Alaska Natives. *Alaska State
Library*

Alaska. Among his duties, he prepared requisitions for medical supplies for hospitals and 10 schools serving as relief stations, examined applicants for the positions of physician and nurse, and submitted those qualified to the commissioner. He also answered a large number of letters from teachers in the field regarding the treatment and care of the sick.

Following the devastating influenza epidemic of 1918–1919, Governor Thomas Riggs Jr. wrote to Surgeon General Blue requesting the assignment of a PHS officer to serve as health commissioner for the territory while also supervising federal health responsibilities, such as the Bureau of Education program. The Legislature even passed a law permitting payment of a $4.00 per diem to offset the cost of living in Juneau. When Blue was unable to find a suitable officer, the governor approached Krulish directly in April. He declined the post because of family considerations, stating that his wife and child "need the outdoor life and food such as fresh eggs and milk," products then not readily available in Juneau. He offered to assist in times of crisis, however, and recommended several individuals for the job.[16]

Dr. Krulish continued for several more years as a consultant to the Bureau of Education from his post in Port Townsend, Washington. As late as 1922 he was assigned to take temporary charge of the Bureau of Education Hospital at Juneau. He later had several other Indian health-related assignments and also served overseas in Czechoslovakia. He retired from the Commissioned Corps in 1942 after 35 years of active duty and died in 1965 at age 86.[17]

In March 1931 the Bureau of Education turned over its medical program to the Office of Indian Affairs, the Medical Branch of which was already under the direction of a PHS commissioned officer. Almost immediately, the PHS detailed Passed Assistant Surgeon Frank Fellows, then 32 years old, to Juneau to take charge of the medical program for Alaska Natives. Soon after his arrival in Alaska in

September 1931, he set off by steamship, Coast Guard vessel, and airplane to visit remote schools and hospitals in the territory, where he assessed the health status of the Alaska Natives and provided training for teachers. He then made many recommendations designed to make the health program more effective and provide greater emphasis on prevention.[18] One of the most important projects initiated during his tenure was his detailed study of the long-term causes of death among Natives. Fellows clearly recognized the limitations of his data, but his analytical report, which was published in 1934, provided the first significant statistical data on health for the territory and called attention to the burgeoning tuberculosis problem.[19]

In the summer of 1934 Fellows was replaced by another commissioned officer, Dr. Vance B. Murray. He arrived in style, flying his own airplane, which he used to visit all the Alaska Native hospitals and villages with nurses over the next six months. In each community he provided direct care and collected data on disease patterns, but the following March he was unexpectedly transferred to a new assignment outside Alaska.[20]

In August 1935 Dr. J. F. van Ackeren replaced him and also took it upon himself to visit all the field posts within the territory, although this time using public transportation. In August 1936 he testified before a Senate committee investigating Indian affairs in Alaska, providing detailed information on health services and disease problems and giving special emphasis to Fellows's report on tuberculosis.[21] In the early summer of 1937 he accompanied Dr. James G. Townsend, then the national Director of Health for the Office of Indian Affairs, on a tour of all the hospitals in Alaska except the one at Unalaska.[22]

The war years, as previously noted, were hard times for support of efforts to improve the health of Alaska Natives, but soon after the war the program had an infusion of new money and staff. Senior Assistant Surgeon Rudolph Haas, a reserve officer, was assigned to Alaska as a tuberculosis specialist in the spring of 1945, spending his mornings at the ANS Hospital at Juneau and his afternoons at the Territorial Health Department. One of his early tasks was to draft a comprehensive strategy for the control of tuberculosis among Alaska Natives.[23] The same month his report was published, he became director of the first postwar sanatorium at Skagway, a rambling former army hospital. Dr. Haas, an orthodox Jew whose father had died in a concentration camp, was described by the staff as "dedicated to his profession, kind and considerate to all." He did his best for the faltering hospital, but left in September 1947 to return to his practice in Portland, Maine.[24]

Following the war the PHS took a much greater interest than before in the health programs for Native Americans. With the departure of Dr. Edgar Norris in 1946, Dr. James A. Smith, also a PHS officer, became Medical Director of the ANS. Among the areas of special concern at this time were dental health, vital statistics, tuberculosis, staff training, and the development of comprehensive health programs. A number of other PHS physicians, dentists, and nurses were detailed to the BIA in FY1945.[25]

In 1946 a 25-year-old, newly minted commissioned officer named Erwin Stuart Rabeau, always known as "Stu," arrived in Kotzebue. In the words of his initial PHS interviewer, he was described as a "neat appearing, rather cocky individual" who wished to serve his country and felt that the PHS was "a good organization to be identified with."[26] He spent the next eleven years in the Arctic, sometimes as the only physician north of Fairbanks. His primary assignment was as Medical Officer-in-Charge of the 45-bed BIA hospital at Kotzebue, but for periods of up to a few years during this time he also had administrative and medical responsibility for the 32-bed hospital at Tanana and the 12-bed hospital at Barrow. Although he had had only limited clinical training during his wartime-accelerated program, he often undertook necessary surgical procedures under the rather primitive operating room conditions at these

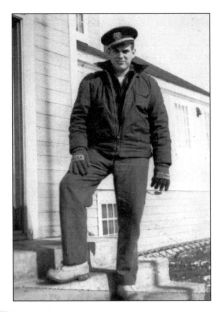

Figure 16. E. S. Rabeau, on the steps of the Kotzebue Hospital, 1950s.
Courtesy of Mary Ann Rabeau

hospitals. Much of his time was spent traveling by small aircraft and dog team not only to the surrounding villages, but also to remote areas such as Little Diomede Island and St. Lawrence Island.

Dr. Rabeau always felt that one of his major accomplishments in bush Alaska was the development of the "radio medical traffic," still known as "radio call" even though it now makes use of satellite telephones. Although he was not the first to use short-wave radio in this way, Rabeau developed and extended the idea of a daily radio consultation, or "sched," with the school teachers, usually beginning at 6:00 PM and extending for several hours. Since the radios of the day were "open band" and there fewer distractions, nearly all those with a short-wave receiver tuned in to find out the interesting medical stories of the day in their neighborhood, and as a by-product learned much about caring for their own common health problems. As a result of his medical skills, his travels, and the radio medical traffic, Rabeau became one of the best known individuals in northern Alaska.

Some idea of the health conditions in Kotzebue during his time there may be gleaned from a report prepared by a visiting medical team from the American Medical Association in 1947:

> Dr. Rabeau at the A N S Hospital at Kotzebue had compiled some decidedly interesting statistics from his records. Kotzebue is a village of 1,200 persons, all Eskimos. For a period of four and one-half years the death rate in this community was 3,600 per hundred thousand. Of these deaths, 54.7 per cent were directly the result of tuberculosis, the diagnosis having been proved by autopsy in over half the cases. . . . In a period of seventeen months he cared for 40 patients with tuberculous meningitis. It was his opinion that 25 per cent of all the natives in the community which he served had open tuberculosis. . . . He further estimated that an additional 35 per cent of the natives had what he would be willing to classify as arrested tuberculosis.[27]

Tuberculosis was clearly the major killer in this era, and in the decade to follow Rabeau was involved in some major developments in the care and prevention of the disease. He was one of the first physicians in Alaska to treat tuberculous cervical lymphadenitis, or scrofula, with the new drug streptomycin, using it in 1948 in a few patients who could afford to purchase it.[28] In the early 1950s he regularly assisted Dr. Philip Moore in major bone-grafting operations at Kotzebue. Moore, Chief of the Territorial Orthopedic Hospital at Mt. Edgecumbe, had developed a technique for transporting frozen bone using dry ice and a special container, allowing him to undertake complex reconstructive surgery for bone and joint tuberculosis in the field.[29] Rabeau, in cooperation with the program of the Alaska Department of Health, also became involved in the use of BCG to prevent tuberculosis.[30]

After eleven years of exhausting but exhilarating work in the Arctic, Rabeau came in from the cold and was assigned as Deputy Medical Officer-in-Charge of the Alaska Area as well as clinical director at the new 400-bed tuberculosis hospital at Anchorage. Additional responsibilities included contract medical care and the supervision of the six other Alaska Native Health Service hospitals at Mt. Edgecumbe, Bethel, Kanakanak, Kotzebue, Tanana, and Barrow. While in Anchorage, he enthusiastically fostered the idea, which he had pioneered in Kotzebue, of having the physicians in the hospitals travel on a regular basis to the Native villages in their service area to provide consultation, case finding, physical examinations, health education, and preventive care. During his tenure the hospital also began an active outpatient clinic and provided specialist consultants to the bush hospitals.

After MPH training in 1960–1961, Rabeau became Indian Health Area Director in Aberdeen, South Dakota. In 1963 he went to Washington as deputy director of the Division of Indian Health and the following year became director at the grade of Assistant Surgeon General. After five years he moved to Tucson, Arizona, as director of the research and development program of the Indian Health Service (as it was then called), where he was responsible for promoting many innovations in health care delivery, especially a Community Health Representative Program and a computerized record system known as the Patient Care Information System, later adopted throughout the IHS. After 35 years as a commissioned officer, he retired in 1981 and returned to Alaska as director of the state Division of Public Health, where he died in office in 1984.[31]

A notable colleague of Rabeau's in northern Alaska was Dr. Robert Lathrop, a dentist who began his Alaskan career in 1948 on the Territorial Health Department's ship M/V *Hygiene* and later transferred to the M/S *Health*. In 1950 he left the ship at Point Hope in northern Alaska and remained there with his wife, living for a year in a Native sod house and subsisting on seals and other Eskimo foods. After a dental refresher course in Michigan in 1952–1953, he returned to Barrow as a dentist for the Bureau of Indian Affairs. When he was transferred to Kotzebue later that year, he and his wife drove a dog team for six weeks in the dead of winter from Barrow to Kotzebue, stopping at villages along the way to provide dental services. He remained at Kotzebue until 1964, joining the Commissioned Corps in 1963. During his subsequent PHS career he served as Area Dental Officer in the Aberdeen area, and, following further public health training, worked at IHS headquarters. He retired in 1975 and now lives in Anchorage.

Chapter 7
The Division of Indian Health/
Indian Health Service in Alaska

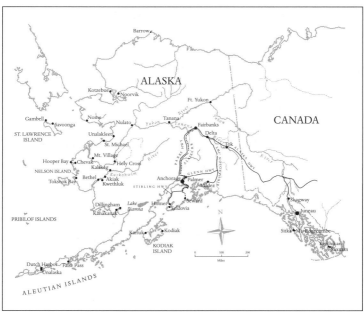

Prior to 1955 various PHS programs in Alaska had a great impact on the health of the people of the territory, but the numbers of officers involved were quite limited, probably no more than a dozen or two at any one time. In contrast, over the next few decades the number of PHS officers and other direct employees of the service in Alaska ranged from a few

Figure 17. Map of Alaska.

hundred to close to 2,000. This change took place when the PHS, as the result of many pressures from without, and not a little resistance from within, took over all health functions and facilities of the Bureau of Indian Affairs on a nationwide scale on July 1, 1955, following passage of PL83-568 by Congress in August 1954. The new administrative unit, initially known as the Division of Indian Health (DIH), was renamed the Indian Health Service (IHS) in 1969. Assistant Surgeon General James R. Shaw, who had headed the BIA medical program while on detail since 1952, became the director of the new agency.[1]

The program in Alaska at the time of the transfer included eight hospitals, located at Anchorage, Mt. Edgecumbe, Juneau, Bethel, Kotzebue, Kanakanak, Tanana, and Barrow. With the exception of the relatively new facilities at Mt. Edgecumbe (1950), Anchorage (1953), and Bethel (1954), these hospitals were of wood frame construction and at least 25 years old. The Juneau hospital was an ancient relic, dating from 1916. Most had totally inadequate facilities for outpatient care.

The medical program at that time served approximately 37,000 Alaska Natives. The principal health problem was still tuberculosis, the prevalence of which, however, was already beginning to decline because of the vigorous program of case-finding, use of BCG, and hospitalization that was begun in 1945 and led by the Alaska Department of Health. Most illness and a third of the deaths were still from infectious diseases that could be prevented by modern control measures. Injuries remained a significant cause of disability and death. The mean age at death for Alaska Natives was 39, compared to 62 in the total US population. Some 41 percent of deaths were in children below the age of four, compared to 7 percent in the US population.[2]

The change in leadership brought an infusion of new ideas, new faces, and the resources of the largest health agency of the US Government. Early priorities of the DIH were to augment and improve medical staffing, outpatient care, support staff, and maintenance. Increased attention to field health services, including public health nursing and sanitation, were also important initiatives. Programs for training of Alaska Natives as practical nurses, dental assistants, and sanitation aides, all begun under BIA, were strengthened.[3]

In Alaska Dr. Theodore E. Hynson, who had been on detail as Medical Director of the Alaska Native Service since November 1953, became the new Area Director in Juneau and the health program was renamed the Alaska Native Health Service. In addition to the post of Area Director PHS commissioned officers soon took over most of the principal professional jobs at the supervisory level, including those of Area Nurse Officer, Area Dental Officer, and Area Pharmacy Officer. Most were career officers who had been working in the Division of Hospitals (Marine Hospitals) or engaging in other clinical activities. The position of Area Executive Officer was added and filled by either a non-physician commissioned officer or a Civil Service employee with experience in hospital administration.

After a period of realignment, a new sense of mission and an expanding vision of comprehensive health care evolved, helped along by better planning, the availability of more health-related technical resources, and increasing budgets. Appropriations remained lean, however, in light of the job to be done, and over the next few decades the staff continued to work under very difficult conditions.

Before 1955 PHS officers who worked in Alaska were for the most part solitary, scattered, and independent of each other. They had little daily interaction with other professionals of their kind and, since Washington was far away and communications sometimes uncertain, they had little sense of community or of membership in the larger organization that was the US Public Health Service.[4] With the coming of the Division of Indian Health, however, PHS officers in Alaska for the first time worked together in numbers with colleagues of their own profession and under the immediate supervision of other commissioned officers.

Dr. Hynson left his post in April 1957 and was replaced temporarily by C. J. Makinen, who remained as Acting Area Director until Dr. Joseph A. Gallagher took over in September of that year. Gallagher was a Regular Corps officer who had come to Alaska in July 1956 as the first PHS Medical Officer-in-Charge (MOC) of the Anchorage Hospital, at that time still primarily a tuberculosis sanatorium. His previous assignment had been as Clinical Director of the PHS Hospital at Staten Island, the largest of the marine hospitals. The Area Office moved from Juneau to Anchorage in 1957 in order to bring it to the center of Native health-related activities, and from that time until his departure for DIH headquarters in July 1959, Gallagher served as both Area Director and MOC of the hospital.

He in turn was replaced by Dr. Kazumi Kasuga, a tuberculosis specialist who had for some years served as clinical director and later Medical Officer-in-Charge at the Tacoma Indian Sanatorium, where many Alaskan tuberculosis patients were still being treated. That year the duties of hospital director were separated from those of the Area Director and, in October 1959, Dr. James A. Hunter, who had served with the Coast Guard in Antarctica, the PHS Hospital at Detroit, and the Federal Prison system, arrived to take over as MOC of the hospital.[5]

A significant change in these early PHS years was the way in which physicians and other professional staff were recruited. This had been a gnawing problem for the BIA, since pay scales and benefits were poor, the posts isolated, and there was little professional supervision or support. From 1955 until the abolition of the draft in 1973, however, young health professionals who had been deferred for study could serve their two-year military commitment in the PHS Commissioned Corps. Some chose the DIH in Alaska for a brief adventure in another world, others came with the thought of settling in Alaska after two years,[6] and a few even came with the intention of making the PHS a career, preferably in Alaska. On the other hand, many of those assigned to Alaska came with the strong anti-government bias characteristic of the era and not a few left with an even stronger aversion after two years of heavy responsibility, relatively low pay, and what they perceived as a lack of support from higher administrative levels.

Previous PHS activities in Alaska had involved primarily physicians, although a few dentists and sanitary engineers (as they were then called) also saw duty with the prewar Territorial Health Department. The new DIH program, however, included professionals from many disciplines. The dental program expanded rapidly both at Anchorage and at the field hospitals and virtually all dentists were commissioned officers. Gradually, too, professional pharmacists, also commissioned officers, were assigned to each of the hospitals. Only a few commissioned nurses were to be found in the earlier years, and those served primarily in administrative and supervisory positions. A scattering of other categories also appeared for the first time, primarily at the Anchorage hospital, including physical therapists, dietitians, and health services officers. In the earlier years, most of the officers in the field hospitals were members of the short-term reserve fulfilling their military obligation, whereas the Area consultants tended to be Regular Corps officers.

A particular onus was placed on the medical officers. Most were young, bright, and energetic, although trained only through the level of internship before being drafted. In the more remote areas, especially, they were thrust into a different cultural environment, perhaps for the first time, with heavy clinical responsibilities. Some were additionally burdened with the unwelcome job of administrative direction of the facility as Medical Officer-in-Charge, or as the post was called after 1963, Service Unit Director (SUD). Most had no experience in management and felt their clinical training was being wasted on administrative tasks.

These young doctors were often functioning well beyond their level of clinical training, especially in complex obstetrical cases, major trauma, or acute abdominal conditions. In surgical cases they used IV pentobarbital, opendrop ether, and spinal anesthetics, and were dependent on an agonizing preparation time with the textbooks before the actual operation. Most had no special training in pediatrics, although half or more of the Alaska Native population was under age 15. Some of the most difficult problems, indeed, were seen in low birth weight newborns or in infants with life-threatening infections, such as meningitis, lobar pneumonia, or severe diarrhea. Tuberculosis was still a major threat, though most physicians had had little or no training in how to deal with it.

Depending on the size of the hospital, each doctor had to take call every two to five nights and weekends throughout the year. Most night and weekend call was exhausting, with numerous outpatient visits punctuated by a few true emergencies, not to mention the inevitable obstetrical deliveries and problems on the wards. Hospital equipment was often antiquated, with the administrative replacement process both glacial and byzantine. Supplies had to be strictly conserved and only drugs from a basic formulary could be prescribed. On nights and weekends the doctor often took his own x-rays, which he then developed and interpreted himself. He also performed urinalyses, white counts, and hematocrits, plated his own cultures, and stained smears and read them. On occasion he performed autopsies unassisted, sometimes for the benefit of the State Troopers.

The daily radio "sched" could last for several hours, and from time to time additional emergency calls interrupted the doctor's routine tasks or hard-won leisure hours. On the radio, physicians were called upon to diagnose and treat serious trauma and illness based on the description by a medically untrained teacher or aide, without the

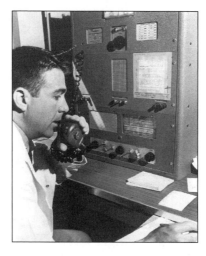

Figure 18. Dr. Jay Keefer conducting radio medical traffic at Bethel, ca. 1962. *PHS photo*

benefit of examining the patient and with little scope for treatment beyond basic antibiotics and aspirin. Patient transportation funds were strictly limited to life-threatening emergencies.

In 1960 a new village clinic program was undertaken in Alaska, due at least in part to the efforts of Dr. Rabeau, who was then Deputy Area Director in Anchorage. This program, dating off and on back to 1907, had been carried out under the auspices of the Bureau of Education and the Bureau of Indian Affairs and had both promoters and detractors. Now, however, the purpose and scheduling of the visits were defined more clearly. The new policy emphasized preventive health services, including immunizations and the examination of schoolchildren, and also provided for case-finding and the treatment of chronic diseases and acute medical problems. Field physicians also learned to extract teeth and perform refractions using trial lenses. By FY1962 physicians, often accompanied by public health nurses or other health workers, conducted regular 1- to-3-day clinics in 25 villages and visited 78 other villages en route. Altogether, 15,696 outpatient visits were reported during 194 village clinics. Over the years to come, this program continued to expand.[7]

On these field trips doctors were called upon to fly in light aircraft through all kinds of weather, spend up to two weeks in a village with no running water, work 12-hour days, and sometimes pass the night in a sleeping bag on a schoolroom table. On occasion the physician traveled between villages by boat, dog-team, snowmobile (after about 1965), and by other means.

These trips could also take a terrible toll. In the winter of 1960 a young PHS medical officer named Stan Edwards was killed in the crash of a light plane on the Alaska Peninsula while en route to a village. His portrait hung for many years at the old Alaska Native Medical Center.[8] Five years later Dr. Charles Hudson and a state public health nurse crashed in a light plane while the pilot was landing on a beach at English Bay (now known as Nanwalek). Both the doctor and the nurse suffered broken vertebrae and had to be evacuated by air to Anchorage.

In December 1968 the Area Director, Dr. John Lee, accompanied by Dr. Francis Raley and Louise Mackin, both from the Alaska Native Medical Center, was involved in a near fatal crash as their Grumman Widgeon was taking off

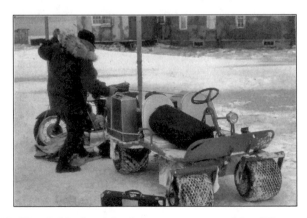

Figure 19. The field physician's gear transported by "Desert Rat" in Platinum, Alaska, 1964. *Photo by author*

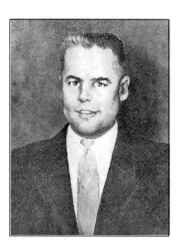

Figure 20. Dr. Stan Edwards, who was killed in a plane crash in 1960. *Photo by author*

from a lake at Pauloff Harbor, in the Aleutians. The wind apparently shifted during take-off and the plane skipped up over a hill at the end of the lake, hit a small ridge, flipped over, and began to burn. Dr. Lee was thrown from the plane and suffered multiple deep cuts on the face and leg. Dr. Raley dragged the unconscious pilot, still buckled in his seat, to safety and then opened the rear door and helped Miss Mackin, who had been hanging upside down in her seat, to safety. The four survivors then scurried behind a nearby hill just in time to see the plane explode. After they returned by skiff to the village, Dr. Raley was asked to examine an eight-year-old boy with a "stomach-ache." The boy was subsequently found to have appendicitis. All five were taken for an eight-hour trip by crab boat to Cold Bay, and from there they flew back to Anchorage. Dr. Raley was later awarded a well-deserved medal for heroism.[9] Every veteran of those years has gripping personal stories to tell about emergency medical missions flown by light plane through marginal weather or darkness.

In 1962 Dr. Holman R. Wherritt arrived to become MOC of the Anchorage hospital, and the following summer he

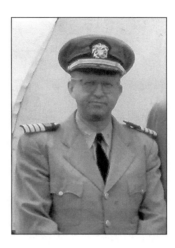

Figure 21. Holman R. Wherritt. *Photo by author*

became Area Director, a post he held until June 1968. Wherritt came with solid experience in Indian health, having served as MOC of the Winnebago Indian Hospital in Nebraska and as Deputy Area Director in the Aberdeen Area.[10] During these years the hospital was gradually metamorphosing into a general hospital, as specialists in pediatrics, obstetrics, orthopedics, ophthalmology, otolaryngology, radiology, and pathology were added to the staff. In the outlying hospitals much emphasis was laid on field health activities, although the staffing remained very sparse. In 1964 the Barrow Hospital had only one physician, while Kanakanak, Tanana, and Kotzebue had two each, and Bethel had four.

Commissioned officers of the Division of Indian Health went into uniform in the summer of 1963. Most of the professional staff, including physicians, dentists, pharmacists, engineers, and sanitarians, were either at the beginning or middle of their two-year military commitment, and the idea of investing money in expensive uniforms for such a short tour of duty was, to say the least, unpopular. Moreover, the Area Office in Anchorage expended little effort to orient new and existing officers about proper dress or military protocol, despite the fact that the city was home to two large military bases. In the field stations, especially, the uniform was often worn incorrectly or not at all. What was particularly troubling to the staff in the field hospitals was that the prescribed uniforms initially made no provision for arctic weather and did not include appropriate footwear, gloves, ear protection, or parkas. The engineers and sanitarians, particularly, deplored the lack of uniforms appropriate for village work. Some of these problems were ultimately addressed by borrowing arctic gear from the Air Force, but the articles matched PHS uniforms poorly and items were not always available or accessible when needed. The IHS went out of uniform again in 1971 and remained that way through the end of the period covered by this survey.

Work conditions such as these took their toll, even on the faithful, and after a few years in the field many officers were burned out and left the service. Others, however, were excited by the life and opportunities in Alaska and applied for DIH-sponsored residencies. Most gladly returned to Alaska, usually as specialists at the Anchorage hospital, where they could continue to hold clinics in the field hospitals. Unlike several Indian Health Area Offices, by the 1970s the Alaska Area had gradually built up a cadre of committed and enthusiastic career officers, some of whom remained in the service for up to 30 years, with no wish ever to leave Alaska.

By 1962 the annual operating budget of the Alaska Area was already twice what it was at the time of transfer. The Alaska Native Health Service was then operating seven hospitals (the Juneau hospital having closed in 1959). The two largest, Anchorage and Mt. Edgecumbe, were called medical centers and each still maintained a tuberculosis unit. The total bed capacity, including the field hospitals, was 900, including 300 for tuberculosis. In addition to the hospitals, the DIH operated school health centers at Mt. Edgecumbe and Wrangell and small clinics at Ketchikan, Fort Yukon, and Nome. During this time the PHS took administrative charge of the small hospitals on St. Paul and St. George Islands in the Pribilof group, far out in the Bering Sea. These facilities had been built and previously maintained by the US Fish and Wildlife Service, which was responsible for most administrative functions on the islands.

The construction budget also expanded dramatically in the years after the transfer. The first new hospital to be built by the PHS in Alaska was a 50-bed facility at Kotzebue, just north of the Arctic Circle, to replace an outmoded hospital dating from 1931. A construction contract was awarded on January 30, 1959, and the hospital was in operation by October 1961.[11] Another new facility built during this era was the 12-bed hospital at Barrow, which was dedicated in November 1965.[12] Building funds were primarily directed

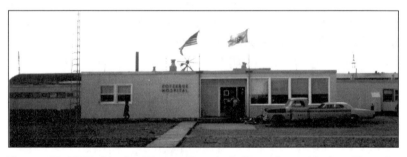

Figure 22. PHS Alaska Native Hospital, Kotzebue, Alaska. *Photo by author*

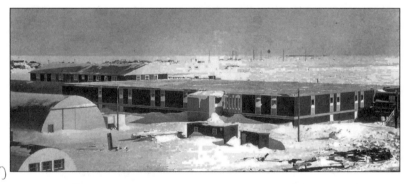

Figure 23. PHS Alaska Native Hospital, Barrow, Alaska. *Photo by author*

to renovations and structural improvements in the older hospitals and to the construction of new staff quarters. The DIH also provided new facilities under PL 85-151, a law that permitted the federal government to furnish financial assistance to community hospitals to expand services to Alaska Natives. The first of these projects was the construction of an outpatient clinic at St. Ann's Hospital in Juneau, and the second provided additional beds at the Ketchikan General Hospital.[13]

Parallel with the expansion of medical services was the growth of the dental program, which was rapidly expanding throughout the area. A dental unit with at least one dentist was located at each of the seven hospitals, the two Pribilof facilities, and at Nome, Fort Yukon, Juneau, and Ketchikan. By 1962 PHS dentists had examined 11,000 patients who made over 25,000 clinic visits. In addition, some dental care was provided through private dentists under contract. A dental laboratory serving all Alaska Natives was located at Mt. Edgecumbe, where there was also a school for training dental assistants. Dental staff teams from the hospitals regularly visited 33 villages, working there from a few days to a month at a time. The greater part of the dental program was directed toward prevention and the treatment of children, although emergency care was given for all ages.[14]

During these years the comprehensiveness of the health program was rapidly expanding in other ways. Pharmacists were first added to the larger hospitals and then ultimately to all hospitals. In the early years the pharmacy at the Anchorage hospital served as the distribution point for all the hospitals and clinics (except Mt. Edgecumbe) and prepackaged all drug orders for field units. Medical social workers were added to several facilities in the early 1960s, as were dietitians at the larger hospitals. In larger hospitals the clinical records were managed by an accredited medical records librarian.

Specialists and consultants, including chief professional officers in dental, nursing, pharmacy, and environmental health, together with a centralized program for finance and budget, general services, personnel, and construction and maintenance, were added to the Area Office. Over the following years offices for program planning, health statistics, systems development, maternal and child health, mental health, nutrition and dietetics, epidemiology, community health, and Native affairs were also added.

Beginning in the early 1960s the DIH gave increased attention to the area of program planning and evaluation throughout the nation. A formalized planning process, with measurable goals and objectives, was established for each Area and each Service Unit. This process was integrated with a system of evaluation so that progress could be assessed and appropriate program changes implemented. This initiative, although unpopular and difficult to implement at the Service Unit level, undoubtedly improved program management.

Another major expansion in the PHS health program in the 1960s was in the area of environmental health. Early PHS efforts in providing direct health care led to the realization that continuing outbreaks of disease could only be controlled if resources were also allocated for making improvements to the environment. This understanding, both in Alaskan villages and Indian reservations in the continental United States, led to the federal Sanitation Facilities Construction Act of 1959 (PL 86-121). This law authorized the PHS to construct sanitary facilities for Indian and Alaska Native communities, including domestic and community water supplies, drainage systems, and facilities for sewage and waste disposal. The DIH was further authorized to make joint arrangements with Alaska Native villages for participation, both in construction costs and in subsequent operation and maintenance of the facilities, as well as to acquire necessary lands, accept contributions, and finally to transfer completed facilities to local authorities for continued operation and maintenance.[15] In 1960 an environmental health unit was established at the Area Office in Anchorage under the direction of James Anderegg. When he transferred to the Alaska Department of Health and Welfare two years later, he was replaced by Kenneth Lauster (1962–1968), followed by Charles Bowman (1968–1971), Ed Jacobsen (1971–1975), and Fred Reif (1975–1979). The staff began by developing guidelines for the new sanitation program. Within two years engineering and sanitarian staff were being hired and funding was allocated for priority construction projects. Many of the initial Alaskan projects involved the development of reliable community water supplies, usually consisting of a new well, simplified water treatment, and a watering point for year-round use. Work first began on planning more complex circulating water distribution systems in larger communities such as Unalakleet and Kotzebue. Other projects, including water exploration, water supply development, and provisions for household water storage and waste disposal, were concurrently developed in smaller communities. In some communities existing water storage and distribution systems and sewerage systems were upgraded or rehabilitated. In

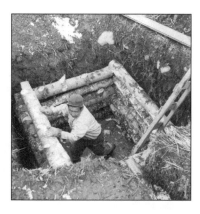

Figure 24. Constructing a seepage pit at English Bay through PL86-121. *Courtesy of James Crum*

others emergency sanitation construction work and the development of refuse collection and disposal facilities were carried out.

The program was soon tied to new federal housing projects in the villages, so that water and sewer service would be available when the houses were completed. Water and sewer improvements were made in dozens of Native communities to serve new housing areas as well as existing homes.

Almost from the beginning of this period of emphasis on environmental health, a PHS sanitarian was assigned to the Area Office, and over the following years others joined the staff and were placed at the field hospitals. Among their initial priorities, they were to conduct sporadic surveys in the rural Alaskan communities, provide some assistance to meet glaring deficiencies, and develop studies of the interrelationship of environmental health improvements, water supply, waste disposal, and housing. Much of this work was done in cooperation with the Alaska Department of Health and Welfare. The sanitarians worked closely with the Sanitation Aide Program, a program in which villagers were trained to teach and demonstrate improved methods of disinfecting water, disposing of waste, and improving home sanitation. These local workers then transmitted the advice and recommendations of the health professionals in a manner that met the values and goals of the local Alaska Native people. As some of the original aides retired, they were replaced with workers who trained villagers as water and sewer operators and conducted environmental health surveys.

During the late 1960s the environmental health program strengthened its relationship with the Alaska state government as various state agencies became involved in funding rural Alaskan sanitation programs. The IHS, under the authority of PL 86-121, continued throughout the 1970s to be a major player in improving sanitation conditions in rural

Alaska in order to lower environmental health-related diseases.[16]

Several other PHS programs operated in close cooperation with other health agencies. Most public health nurse functions and the sanitation aide program in bush areas were carried out by the Alaska Department of Health and Welfare under contract with DIH. A coordinated nutrition education program was also a joint project of DIH, the Alaska Department of Health and Welfare, and the Bureau of Indian Affairs. The Alaska Native Health Service also jointly sponsored several significant research projects in cooperation with the Arctic Health Research Center (see next chapter).[17]

On March 27, 1964, the great Good Friday earthquake struck Alaska, causing vast geological upheavals and tsunamis but little loss of life. Many buildings in downtown Anchorage suffered substantial harm, but the PHS Alaska Native Hospital located there, though badly shaken, escaped with only minor structural damage and no serious injuries to either patients or staff. The bluff behind the hospital fell away, however, initiating a seemingly endless struggle between Anchorage and Washington to build a replacement hospital, a quest that ended more than three decades later with the opening of the new Alaska Native Medical Center in 1997. In the immediate aftermath of the quake, the hospital staff issued warm clothing to its own patients, set up an emergency sanitation system for the hospital, offered assistance to other area hospitals, housed the homeless, and joined city health officials in offering immunization clinics. In the days that followed, many villagers from inundated communities on Kodiak Island were air-evacuated to Anchorage, where they were housed in a school. PHS physicians screened all these evacuees and offered any needed preventive services or treatment. Other physicians, nurses, and sanitarians were sent out to provide health services in the villages damaged in the quake.[18]

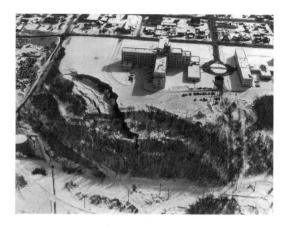

Figure 25. The PHS Alaska Native Hospital at the time of the Great Alaska Earthquake, March 27, 1964. *PHS photo*

A significant milestone in the health program around this time was the development of the Community Health Aide Program. Community health aides were Alaska Natives, chosen by their village leaders, who initiated care for minor injuries and illnesses and reported the more serious cases by radio to the physician at the regional hospital. This role had once been carried out by teachers or missionaries but, beginning in the 1950s, it was gradually taken over by local villagers known as village medical aides, who received on-the-job training by visiting public health nurses and physicians. The first specific training program for them was held at the Kotzebue hospital in 1964 and was followed by a similar program at Bethel in late 1964 and early 1965. These initial efforts were so successful and so well received that an Area-wide training program was funded by Congress in 1968—the Community Health Aide Program, or CHAP. Health aides from all over the state came to Anchorage for what ultimately became a 12-week course of instruction held in several phases. A detailed manual was developed as a reference guide for health aides in the villages. Subsequently, several Native health corporations took over training responsibilities in their own regions.[19]

In July 1968 Dr. John F. Lee became Area Director, the last commissioned officer to hold the post.[20] Lee, trained in surgery and public health, had previously served in the Division of Hospitals, in Ethiopia (with the Peace Corps), and even on board the tall ship USCGC *Eagle* on a cruise to Greenland. His tenure was especially marked by a concerted effort to involve the Alaska Native peoples in the management of their own health services. He also provided leadership in addressing, in a positive manner, controversies that arose with the private medical sector.[21]

Beginning in the late 1960s, Lee had established consumer boards for the state as a whole and for each Service Unit. These boards, selected by Native organizations in the areas served by the hospitals, enabled people to share in the responsibility of improving their health by active participation in the planning, conduct, and evaluation of the health program. During the early 1970s the boards gradually assumed more and more influence in the operations of each Service Unit, aided and supported by the Office of Native Affairs at the Area Office. Consumer participation was also accomplished through contracts with Alaska Native organizations and village councils to provide certain services, such as special health programs and training and employment of community health aides. He was also among the first to place Alaska Natives in positions of authority at the Area level.

In 1978 the Alaska Area Native Health Service, as it was then called, was the Alaska regional program of the Indian Health Service and was serving an estimated 65,000 Alaska Natives living in urban areas and 181 villages. The Area program included eight Service Units: Anchorage (including the Alaska Native Medical Center and the Pribilof hospitals), Barrow, Bethel, Kanakanak, Kotzebue, Norton Sound, Mt. Edgecumbe, and Interior Alaska. Each of these regional units included a hospital (some with one or more satellite clinics) and was responsible for a large geographical area of the state. Each served a largely uniform ethnic community and each had an active health board that played an active part in planning, setting priorities, and program evaluation.

The Area Office administrative structure continued to evolve and now included units in environmental health, program formulation, patient care standards, community health services, construction and maintenance, general services, financial management, and personnel and training. Each Service Unit had greater autonomy than before, although many services, including personnel and financial management, were still centralized. Service Unit Directors were no longer physicians except for the director of the Alaska Native Medical Center, although a few were commissioned officers trained in health services administration. Nearly all physicians, dentists, pharmacists, engineers, sanitarians, and physical therapists remained commissioned officers, as did a few nurses, dietitians, and health services officers. Well over half of the total employees, including both the Area Director and his deputy, were Alaska Natives.

Health care was provided at three levels. Primary care at the village level was in the hands of health practitioners, who visited the village periodically, and community health aides, who had been trained either in Anchorage or by one of the regional health corporations. Clinic-based care was provided by physicians, dentists, physician assistants, nurse practitioners, and other health workers at fixed facilities. The secondary level of care, at the regional hospitals or the Alaska Native Medical Center, included hospitalization for routine illnesses, obstetrical care, minor surgery, and specialist outpatient care. Tertiary care was the province of the Alaska Native Medical Center, where a full range of specialists was available. Sophisticated care not available at ANMC was provided under contract with either private practitioners or hospitals in Anchorage, or occasionally in Seattle or other university centers.[22]

The health status of the Alaska Natives by 1978 was undergoing marked changes. Tuberculosis was no longer a major threat and other infectious diseases were steadily declining in relative importance. Chronic otitis media and its sequelae were nearly absent, but other chronic diseases, notably atherosclerotic heart disease, hypertension, stroke, and cancer, were rapidly gaining ground. Diabetes, once rare, was being increasingly diagnosed. Injuries due to accidents or violence remained a major problem, as was alcohol and tobacco abuse. Mental health problems were becoming more prevalent, in part because of the cultural disruption of urban migration and the loss of a subsistence economly. Overall, the health patterns of the Alaska Natives were approaching those of the general population.

During the period 1955 to 1978 many individuals in the Public Health Service served in Alaska with distinction on both the administrative and the clinical level. One couple with a great impact were the Wilsons, Martha and Joe, who came from the Indian Sanatorium at Tacoma to Mt. Edgecumbe in 1959, she as a tuberculosis specialist and he as a thoracic surgeon. They moved to the Anchorage Hospital in 1961, where she later became Chief of Medicine and he Chief of Surgery. In 1963 Dr. Martha (as she was universally called) became Service Unit Director and over the next eight years led the transition of the hospital from a tuberculosis sanatorium to a general medical and surgical referral hospital, a transformation that was reflected by an official name change in 1965 to the Alaska Native Medical Center. One of her special priorities for the hospital was the provision of prompt specialty consultation and support, including continuing education, for all field hospitals. She also exhibited leadership qualities in the development of special programs for rehabilitation and for the treatment of otitis media. When Robert Fortuine became Director of the Medical Center in 1971, Dr. Martha became Director of Program Development at the Area Office, where she made important contributions in the area of computerized health records

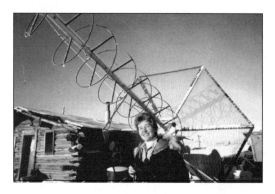

Figure 26. Dr. Martha R. Wilson, with ATS-6 satellite antenna. *PHS photo*

and satellite communications for health, the latter in a project funded in part by the Lister Hill National Center for Biomedical Communication at the National Library of Medicine. Her career was cut short by cancer in 1979.[23] Joe Wilson continued to serve for many years as Chief of Surgery and made important clinical and research contributions in the areas of bronchiectasis and alveolar hydatid disease.

Another individual who made outstanding contributions was Dr. M. Walter Johnson, who began his PHS career in Bethel in the 1950s and later became chief of medicine, tuberculosis control officer, and finally clinical director at the Alaska Native Medical Center. He also played an important part in the development and expansion of the Community Health Aide Program in Alaska and in the development of the Alaska Health Sciences Library (see next chapter).

Although not a commissioned officer, Dr. Gloria K. Park was another physician who dedicated her whole professional life to the Public Health Service and its health program for Alaska Natives. She arrived at the Alaska Native Hospital in 1957 as chief of the new outpatient clinic and remained until her retirement in 1986, serving longer than any other full-time physician. Her special contributions included the fostering of ambulatory care, preventive programs in the field, and the Community Health Aide Program. Several notable clinicians started their careers as Service Unit Directors in the field hospitals and achieved distinction in a clinical specialty, among them Ken Fleshman and Ward Hurlburt (Kanakanak), and Osamu Matsutani (Barrow), in pediatrics, surgery, and psychiatry, respectively. George Wagnon spent many years as a Service Unit Director in Kanakanak, Bethel, and Mt. Edgecumbe. Two other former Service Unit Directors, Charles H. Neilson and Ward Hurlburt, became Deputy Area Directors. One of the most remarkable stories is that of Daniel J. O'Connell, who, though never a Service Unit Director, has remained for well over 20 years as a clinical physician in bush Alaska, serving at Kotzebue, Bethel, Kanakanak, Ketchikan, and Metlakatla. Another was William James, who served well over two decades at the Tanana Hospital and the PHS clinic at Fairbanks. Several clinical physicians began as general medical officers in Alaska in the 1960s and 1970s, then, after Service-sponsored residencies came back for long-term assignments as specialists at Anchorage or Mt. Edgecumbe. These included George Brenneman, John Christopherson, Ken Petersen, and Lee M. Schmidt in pediatrics, Clyde Farson in ophthalmology, Dudley Weider in otolaryngology, Brian McMahon in internal medicine, and Anne Lanier in epidemiology. Many other dedicated specialists served the hospitals well over a long period, notably David Dolese, a general surgeon who came to Anchorage in 1961 and remained there until his retirement over 20 years later, Dr. David W. Templin, who came to ANMC in 1969 and still serves as an active consultant in rheumatology, and David Barrett, who has served the hospital for more nearly three decades as an internist or as Chief of Medicine.

A few long-time clinical physicians also found time to make distinctive and significant contributions to research, particularly Joseph Wilson in echinococcal disease, Anne

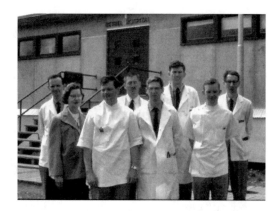

Figure 27. Professional staff at PHS Alaska Native Hospital, Bethel, Alaska, 1965. L-R Robert Fortuine (SUD), Katherine Holland (Director of Nursing), Richard Scott (dentist), Daniel J. O'Connell (physician), Lee M. Schmidt (physician), Eugene Trout (physician), David Heimke (pharmacist), and George Brenneman (physician). All but Scott, Trout, and Heimke became career officers. *Photo by author*

Lanier in cancer epidemiology, Brian McMahon in liver disease, David Templin in rheumatic diseases, and George Brenneman and Ken Petersen in pediatric infectious diseases.

In the early years of the DIH, commissioned officer physicians generally served in the top administrative positions at each Service Unit, as Medical Officers-in-Charge. After 1963 they were known as Service Unit Directors, and each was assisted by an administrative officer. In the mid-1960s, however, a new DIH policy allowed non-physicians to become SUDs. Arthur C. Willman began his Alaska career as a pharmacist at Kotzebue in January 1962, and over the following two years gradually took on the responsibilities of hospital administrative officer. In 1966 he became the first non-physician to be sponsored by DIH for postgraduate administrative training, ultimately obtaining a Master of Science in Administrative Medicine degree at Columbia. Following three years as Deputy Service Unit Director at the Gallup Indian Medical Center, he returned to Alaska in 1971 as hospital director and later Service Unit

Director at the Mt. Edgecumbe Hospital. Two other Health Services Officers with long service in Alaska were James Armbrust, who began as Service Unit Director at Tanana, and Banks Warden, who was for several years the Service Unit Director at Kanakanak.[24]

Many other career officers served with distinction and remained with the program in some capacity until retirement and sometimes beyond. Among many other non-physicians who should be mentioned for their long and distinguished service in Alaska are Douglas Smole and Tom Kovaleski in dentistry, Robert Baus in physical therapy, and Roger Dinwiddie, James Hayes, and Emil Cekada in pharmacy.

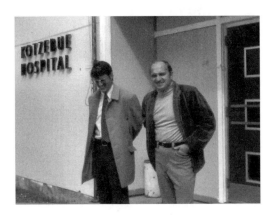

Figure 28. Banks Warden and Arthur Willman outside Kotzebue Hospital, ca 1976. *Photo by author*

Chapter 8
Northern Health Research

arlier examples of PHS health-related research in Alaska have already been cited, namely Frank Fellows's study of Alaska mortality rates in the early 1930s and the long-term study of BCG in the 1930s and 1940s by Dr. Joseph Aronson of the Phipps Institute, supported financially by the PHS. In FY1949 the National Institute of Health largely funded a small study on the use of streptomycin in bone and joint tuberculosis at the Mt. Edgecumbe Orthopedic Hospital and in pulmonary tuberculosis at the Seward Sanatorium.[1] Since 1949, however, biomedical research in Alaska has largely been the province of two PHS agencies, the Arctic Health Research Center (AHRC) and the Centers for Disease Control and Prevention (CDC).

The need for a research program to study the special health problems of northern climates was recognized as early as 1942, and by 1947 the PHS was formulating plans to establish an Arctic Institute of Health to study the relation of heath to the special conditions found in northern latitudes.[2] That summer a visiting AMA survey team considered the issue and later recommended to Congress that federal funds be provided to establish an Arctic Institute on the university campus at Fairbanks for the study of health, sanitation, nutrition, construction, food, and clothing in relation to northern climates.[3]

The so-called Alaska Health Grant of $1,150,000, appropriated by Congress in 1948 and channeled through PHS, called for increased cooperation between the PHS and the Alaska Department of Health (ADH) "in activities necessary in the investigation, prevention, treatment, and control of diseases, and the establishment and maintenance of health and sanitation services." Although most of these funds were thus designated for the expansion of ADH services, $223,000 was allocated to begin a research program in a new health research station to be established in Anchorage. The first director was Dr. Jack C. Haldeman, an experienced PHS officer who had first come to Alaska in July 1938 as a tuberculosis clinician and acting territorial epidemiologist.[4]

Haldeman set up temporary headquarters in mid-town Anchorage during the summer of 1948, but within a couple of years the program had moved to much more satisfactory surroundings in a new apartment building at 6th and K Streets. The building included approximately 9,000 square feet which was soon converted for laboratory bench research, complete with stainless-steel laboratory furniture, modern scientific equipment, incubator space, walk-in refrigeration, and deep-freeze units. Supporting services included space for the care and breeding of small laboratory animals, preparation of biological media, and dishwashing. The administrative staff was located in a building next door. Ultimately, an entomological laboratory and shop, instrument shop, arctic animal house, and storage facilities were established elsewhere in the city.

In a summary of activities written a few years later, Haldeman described the program approach of what came to be known as the Arctic Health Research Center, located administratively under the PHS Bureau of State Services:

> Our pattern of organization differs from that of many research activities in Alaska in that the work is largely carried out by a staff resident in the Territory devoting full time to investigation. Anchorage was selected as a base of operations, since it is a principal transportation center and offered the best opportunity for renting and

converting suitable space for laboratory facilities as well as for obtaining housing for our personnel. . . . The recruitment of our professional staff has not been as difficult as anticipated, possibly because of the unparalleled opportunities for research in the area.[5]

Haldeman also recognized the importance of good staff living conditions and good administrative direction, especially those related to the acquisition of supplies and equipment, rental of space, contracts, and personnel actions. From the beginning, AHRC staff offered "Stateside colleagues" the benefit of their experience and knowledge of Alaska to assist them in preparing for scientific field trips to remote areas. They also offered them consultative services and, within physical limits, the use of the Anchorage facilities.

By 1951 AHRC had four experienced scientists working in arctic physiology who were studying problems related to the natural adjustments of animals to cold, using measurements of respiratory metabolism, body and skin temperature, and oxygen consumption. Their laboratory included a cold test room providing temperatures ranging from +35° C to -55° C.

The studies of the Nutrition and Biochemistry Section were carried out by three biochemists and one physiologist. Among their activities were food analysis, clinical and enzyme chemistry, and tissue respiration studies. Facilities were also available for carrying out experiments in small animal nutrition.

The Zoonotic Disease Section included three scientists with collective experience in veterinary medicine, general parasitology, helminth taxonomy, and mammalian taxonomy and pathology. The laboratory was equipped with autopsy facilities and apparatus necessary for parasitological investigations, a rotary and a freezing microtome, aquaria, and a dark room for macro- and microphotography.

An entomologist, aquatic biologist, entomological engineer, and insect control specialist worked in the

Entomological Section. Their resources included an insect collection and an entomological shop with the equipment necessary for the development and construction of special types of apparatus for Alaskan insect control operations. Two bacteriological laboratories were maintained, one devoted to the study of water supply and sewage disposal and the other to the study of infectious diseases. Space was also provided for a branch laboratory of the Alaska Department of Health, which made available specimens for analysis. Engineers engaged in environmental sanitation studies had available a pilot well and experimental septic tank installations located on the grounds of the University of Alaska, as well as facilities operated by the city of Fairbanks and the Air Force at Ladd Field.

Since no libraries relating to the biomedical sciences were then available in Alaska, the development of a research library was considered an essential task. Before long AHRC was receiving and circulating some 200 scientific periodicals. The library staff was also very successful in promptly obtaining many needed publications, microfilms, and photostats.[6]

The AHRC facility was also equipped with an instrument shop equipped to do all ordinary metalwork such as turning, cutting, and welding, small wood and plastic work, and sheet metalwork of limited size. It also maintained an animal house, located on the outskirts of Anchorage, with a collection of native animals, including black bears, marmots, ground squirrels, red and blue foxes, tree squirrels, porcupines, weasels, geese, conies, Eskimo dogs, and even Norway rats living under conditions approximating their natural habitat.[7]

The original station in Anchorage was just the beginning. In October 1948 the Regents of the University of Alaska donated a campus site for the new institute. In January 1949 the federal budget included the generous figure of $7,350,000 for FY1950 to establish a major new "Arctic Institute of Health" at the university. This research center provided laboratories, coordination of effort to avoid duplication, and an academic environment for health researchers in the territory. When the Bureau of the Budget tried to place a lower priority on the project, Alaska Governor Ernest Gruening wrote a detailed rebuttal setting forth the many advantages of such a research program and facility.[8]

When investigative activities were first undertaken, the almost complete lack of information pertaining to Alaska in the various scientific fields required the staff to start from scratch, painstakingly collecting and sifting the few available data and making on-the-spot surveys. Limited resources made it necessary to concentrate in areas with the greatest immediate health impact. The staff endeavored to strike a balance between basic research, such as biochemistry and physiology, and applied research, such as studies in water supply, waste disposal, and insect control. In addition, certain "background" investigations were undertaken that included studies of animal-borne diseases transmissible to man and the distribution and life habits of biting insects.[9]

The institute was thus conceived as an independent, self-sustaining establishment, with its research program planned and developed with sufficient scope to embrace all aspects of medicine and biology relating to human existence in an arctic environment, including problems of housing, food, clothing, sanitation, microbiology, entomology, and disease control investigation.[10] Its primary task would be to coordinate all the sporadic research efforts of the past and to provide year-round and cumulative data on arctic-related health issues.

In 1951 Dr. Haldeman was replaced by Dr. E. T. Blomquist, who had been the Assistant Chief of the PHS Division of Tuberculosis Control in Washington, D.C.[11] He in turn was replaced by Dr. A. B. Colyar a few years later, and in 1969 Dr. Edward M. Scott became the director. These four individuals presided over a far-ranging research program, some aspects of which are briefly described below.

By 1968 AHRC scientists and physicians had published some 563 papers that greatly expanded our knowledge of the complex relationships of the arctic environment to the health of its peoples.[12]

In the environmental area the center studied the design of existing water supply and waste disposal systems, housing, and cold weather clothing in the Arctic and developed several practical and innovative designs of its own. The engineers also addressed the effects of permafrost and the long winter freeze on water storage and supply and on waste disposal. In one study they attempted to trace pollution through the introduction of bacterial agents and chemical indicators into ground water supplies. In another they examined the effect of freezing on water supply and sewage disposal by drilling an experimental well through 70 feet of permafrost and demonstrating that the rate of pumping influenced freezing. Beginning about 1955, in cooperation with the Alaska Department of Health and Welfare and the Alaska Native Health Service, the section began to direct its efforts toward the improvement of sanitary conditions in small, isolated villages. As part of an experimental sanitation program carried out in a few isolated villages to demonstrate the practicability of developing water supplies under PL86-121, the staff constructed with the help of villagers the first experimental well ever developed in a permafrost area. Another project involved the construction of several experimental houses in Native villages. By 1960 the section had achieved the first successful winter-long operation of an airlock system to prevent freezing of water supply lines during intervals between pumping periods. In other studies they developed a windmill-driven generator to provide heat for thawing, sewage stabilization lagoons, and experimental recirculating waste treatment units. After the 1964 earthquake the Environmental Health Section assisted in the design and reconstruction of some of the villages destroyed by tsunamis.

The Physiology Section carried out field studies on the adaptation of animals and man to the arctic environment, some of them in collaboration with scientists from Canada, Norway, Sweden, and England, as well as with those of the University of Alaska and the US Air Force. Arctic mammals and birds were studied in order to determine the processes, including metabolic rate, hibernation, and circulation in exposed tissues, that enabled them to live successfully in temperatures at which unadapted animals and their tissues ceased to function.

The Zoonotic Disease Section, under the able leadership of veterinary officer Dr. Robert L. Rausch, carried out extensive studies on animal carcasses obtained from hunters and trappers to determine the distribution and life cycle of northern parasites, particularly *Trichinella*, two species of *Echinococcus*, and fish tapeworm, as well as studies of rabies, tularemia, brucellosis, and encephalitis. Several new species of arctic parasites were identified and described, and the life cycles of others were established in detail for the first time. In one study they showed that about 30 percent of the Eskimos have a positive intradermal reaction to trichinosis. The section also successfully carried out both rabies control measures and a canine distemper vaccination program in the Arctic, and promoted a ban on the importation of dogs from St. Lawrence Island to the mainland because of the danger of spreading *Echinococcus multilocularis* disease.

The Entomology Section identified and surveyed Alaskan biting insects and determined their life cycles, breeding habits, and distribution as a basis for the development of practical control measures. Newer forms and improved methods of DDT spraying were found to be effective against black fly larvae in Alaskan streams without appreciable damage to fish or fish food. Widespread application of an aerosol spray unit that was developed in 1949 for the control of adult insects demonstrated the effectiveness and economic value of this device in Alaska.

The Biochemistry and Nutrition Section, headed for many years by Dr. Edward M. Scott, conducted a major dietary survey of the Alaska Natives that included hemoglobin studies, glucose, vitamin A, and cholesterol determinations, and estimates of the nutritional content and value of Alaska Native foods. These findings were then correlated with data on the prevalence of coronary atherosclerosis. Research was especially directed toward identifying biochemical changes and deviations in nutritional requirements resulting from living in an arctic environment. These extensive food intake and analysis studies greatly clarified the nutritional status of the Eskimos. Later studies involved village surveys for anemia and a search for diabetes mellitus among the Eskimos. This section also conducted many genetic studies that resulted in the identification of several conditions with a high prevalence among Eskimos, including methemoglobinemia, adrenogenital syndrome, and cholinesterase deficiency. Kuskokwim disease, a new form of congenital arthrogryposis, was identified in Yup'ik Eskimos in the early 1970s.

The Epidemiology Section investigated many outbreaks of acute disease, including trichinosis, influenza, pediatric respiratory disease, measles, mumps, rubella, and poliomyelitis. A major byproduct of these studies, developed in cooperation with the PHS Rocky Mountain Laboratory in Montana, was the gradual accumulation of a valuable frozen serum bank that was useful for the detection and distribution of various antibodies in the Alaska Native population. A significant undertaking in the 1950s, in conjunction with the Alaska Department of Health and Welfare, was the McGrath Project, in which an Indian town was surveyed for eye, ear, nose, and throat diseases, as well as for tuberculosis status and dental disease. A particularly important series of investigations, developed from an infant morbidity and mortality cohort investigation that was initiated in the Bethel area in 1962 and continued for decades, yielded significant information not only on disease patterns but on such issues as growth and development, deafness, and learning disabilities. Later, field trials of new measles and rubella vaccines were initiated among the highly susceptible Alaska Natives. Another major field of interest was the prevalence of enteric pathogens, and a survey of several villages was carried out in cooperation with the Harvard School of Public Health and the Armed Forces Board of Epidemiology. Among the principal investigators who made their mark in this era were James Maynard, who later headed the CDC Hepatitis Laboratory, and Jacob Brody, who went on to a distinguished career at NIH.

A notable feature of the AHRC was its close association with other health agencies working to solve current and urgent health problems. By all odds the most important research studies of this type were those on ambulatory chemotherapy and INH prophylaxis of tuberculosis. These studies were conceived, designed, and carried out in close cooperation with the Alaska Department of Health, the Alaska Native Service (BIA), and other agencies of the Public Health Service, particularly the Tuberculosis Program. The first, known as the Ambulatory Chemotherapy Program, or ACP, was carried out from 1954 to 1957 in over 70 villages of western, northern, and interior Alaska. They were undertaken at a time when all tuberculosis beds were filled and the territory had a waiting list of nearly 2,000 for hospitalization. The AHRC organized a team of physicians and nurses to survey the population, dispense INH and PAS to patients awaiting hospitalization, and tabulate the results. These results, in fact, were spectacular and before long the hard-won tuberculosis hospitals were being emptied out. A spin-off of this program was a series of papers on the definition and distribution of phlyctenular keratoconjunctivitis (PKC), a related inflammatory eye disease causing much visual loss in Alaska.

Once the program was on a solid footing, the AHRC turned it over to the Department of Health, except in the Yukon-Kuskokwim region, where in 1957 it began a series of studies in the Bethel area, under the able and enthusiastic leadership of Dr. George W. Comstock, to determine the effectiveness of administering INH to prevent tuberculosis. The first round was a double-blind study of INH for those without evidence of active tuberculosis that showed about a 70 percent reduction in the incidence of the disease. The results were so favorable that a second community-wide study was initiated in 1964 to allow those who had received placebo in the first study, plus other members of the community, to enjoy the benefits of the drug.

Collaborative and in-house research continued on a variety of diseases and health conditions of significance to the Alaska Native people. A new AHRC building was finished in the fall of 1966 on the University of Alaska campus in Fairbanks where, over the next few years, the greater part of the program operated in close cooperation with other research units of the university. The Epidemiology Section remained in Anchorage, however, largely because of its need for access to the clinical facilities there, especially at the ANMC.

AHRC officially closed in 1973, the victim of a budget crunch, but the work of the epidemiology unit continued in Anchorage, initially under the direction of the Ecological Investigations Program of the Centers for Disease Control and Prevention. Several of the senior AHRC staff from other sections, notably Edward M. Scott, remained active in research with the new program. This unit later became known as the Alaska Investigations Division of the CDC Bureau of Epidemiology, which established a laboratory facility on the grounds of the Alaska Native Medical Center. In 1980 the name was changed to the Arctic Investigations Laboratory, and later still the Arctic Investigations Program, which continued studies in the areas of infant mortality and

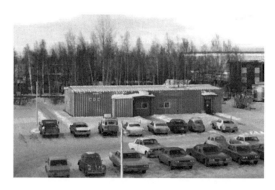

Figure 29. CDC / Arctic Investigations Program building on campus of the old Alaska Native Medical Center, Anchorage. *CDC photo*

infectious diseases of children. A prevention program for streptococcal disease was established and research continued on the causes of meningitis and anemia, the effects of otitis media, hepatitis, genetic and metabolic disorders, the epidemiology of cancer, and food-borne botulism. The CDC program has continued to carry out carefully designed laboratory and epidemiological investigations on pressing health problems specific to the northern regions.

A representative list of research publications and reports by scientists of the Arctic Health Research Center and the Arctic Investigations Program of the CDC can be found in the Appendix.

Epilogue

n this monograph I have presented just a few of the notable accomplishments of the US Public Health Service during its first century in Alaska. In the additional quarter of a century since 1978, the Commissioned Corps of the Public Health Service has continued many of its missions, particularly in Indian Health and in research.

The Commissioned Corps in Alaska probably reached its apogee in the 1960s and 1970s when all but a few of the PHS physicians, dentists, pharmacists, engineers, and sanitarians were commissioned. In the years since about 1980, the number of officers in Alaska has declined significantly, in part because of the end of the doctor draft, but much more so because of the rapid shift from directly operated Alaska health programs to those managed and operated by Native health corporations under authority of the Indian Self-Determination and Educational Assistance Act of 1975. This process was completed when the largest facility in the Indian Health Service, the new Alaska Native Medical Center in Anchorage, was turned over to the Alaska Native Tribal Health Consortium and the Southcentral Foundation in 1999. Although some tribal health authorities continue to recruit and retain commissioned officers, the trend has been for them to seek out applicants for the professional staff and hire them directly. Commissioned officers, however, still fill many key professional and administrative positions in the present health care system for Alaska Natives. They still wear the uniform but are detailed to the appropriate Native health corporation and serve under its supervision.

The Arctic Investigations Program of CDC has pursued its fine tradition of research, particularly in the field of epidemiology of cancer and infectious diseases. It now enjoys new and greatly expanded facilities on the campus of the new Alaska Native Medical Center, where its staff continues to work in close cooperation with the professional staff of the hospital.

The State Department of Health and Social Services, particularly the Division of Public Health, still benefits from many PHS grants, mainly from CDC and NIH. An Epidemic Intelligence Service Officer is regularly assigned to the Epidemiology Section to assist in the investigation of disease outbreaks in the state.

The US Public Health Service has a long and proud tradition in Alaska. In a vast territory with sometimes treacherous weather and huge logistical difficulties, and whose diverse peoples have suffered health problems of unprecedented complexity and severity, officers and employees of the PHS have served on many fronts with skill, courage, enthusiasm, and distinction. Both as individuals and as members of larger units, they have brought initiative, ingenuity, and resourcefulness to the solution of the difficult problems facing them. They have often confronted grave responsibilities beyond their training and experience, while enduring professional and personal isolation, physical danger, long hours, marginal living conditions, and inadequate resources. Their contributions to the better health of all Alaskans have been lasting and significant, and will not soon be forgotten.

Notes

Chapter 1

1. Ralph Chester Williams, *The United States Public Health Service, 1798–1950* (Washington: Commissioned Officers Association of USPHS, 1951); Bess Furman, *A Profile of the United States Public Health Service, 1798–1948* (Bethesda, Md.: US Department of Health, Education and Welfare, National Institutes of Health, National Library of Medicine, 1973), DHEW Publication No. (NIH) 73–369; Fitzhugh Mullan, *Plagues and Politics: The Story of the United States Public Health Service* (New York: Basic Books, 1989).

2. The term "Alaska Natives" refers to the indigenous peoples who often refer to themselves as simply "Natives," a term that is not considered pejorative.

3. A good recent history of Alaska is by Stephen Haycox, entitled *Alaska: An American Colony* (Seattle: University of Washington Press, 2002).

4. For a detailed account of the period before 1900, see the author's *Chills and Fever: Health and Disease in the Early History of Alaska* (Fairbanks: University of Alaska Press, 1989).

5. See the author's *"Must We All Die?" Alaska's Enduring Struggle with Tuberculosis* (Fairbanks: University of Alaska Press, 2005).

6. For further information on Alaska Native health in the early twentieth century, see the author's paper "Health care and the Alaska Native: Some historical perspectives," *Polar Notes, Occasional Publication of the Stefansson Collection* (Dartmouth) XIV (1975): 1–42.

Chapter 2

1. Stephen Hadley Evans, *The United States Coast Guard, 1790–1915: A Definitive History, with a Postscript: 1915–1950* (Annapolis: United States Naval Institute, 1949), 109.

2. Morgan B. Sherwood, *Exploration of Alaska, 1865–1900* (New Haven: Yale University Press, 1965), 120.

3. Ralph Chester Williams, *The United States Public Health Service, 1798–1950* (Washington: Commissioned Officers Association of USPHS, 1951), 412.

4. Throughout this paper, MHS and PHS ranks are given in their original form. Navy equivalents are as follows: Assistant Surgeon = Lieutenant (jg); Passed (or Senior) Assistant Surgeon = Lieutenant; Surgeon = Lieutenant Commander; Senior Surgeon = Commander; Medical Director = Captain; Assistant Surgeon General and Deputy Surgeon General = Rear Admiral (lower and upper grades); Surgeon General = Vice Admiral.

5. George W. Bailey, *Report upon Alaska and its People, United States Revenue-Cutter Service* (Washington: Government Printing Office, 1880), 1–52. White's report is on pages 33–42.

6. Robert White, "Notes on the physical condition of the inhabitants of Alaska," in Bailey, *Report*, 33.

7. The Surgeon General's Report for 1880 states that "one assistant surgeon died from disease probably contracted in the service. The fatal termination was doubtless hastened by the exposures incident to the climate of Alaska and the voyage thither." It seems likely that the officer in question was Dr. White. *Annual Report of the Supervising Surgeon-General of the Marine-Hospital Service of the United States, for the Fiscal Year 1880* (Washington: Government Printing Office, 1880), 24.

8. C. L. Hooper, *Report of the Cruise of the US Revenue-Steamer* Corwin *in the Arctic Ocean, November 1, 1880* (Washington: Government Printing Office, 1881), 39.

9. Healy was of African-American descent, although this fact was not known to his contemporaries.

10. Irving C. Rosse, "Medical and anthropological notes of Alaska." In United States Department of the Treasury, *Cruise of the Revenue Steamer* Corwin *in Alaska and the N. W. Arctic Ocean in 1881 . . . Notes and Memoranda . . . United States Revenue-Cutter Service,* Treasury Document No. 429 (Washington: Government Printing Office, 1883), 19.

11. Rosse, "Medical and anthropological notes," 24.

12. Michael A. Healy, *Report of the Cruise of the Revenue Steamer* Corwin *in the Arctic Ocean in the Year 1885* (Washington: Government Printing Office, 1887), 17.

13. *Annual Report of the Supervising Surgeon-General of the Marine-Hospital Service of the United States for the Fiscal Year 1888* (Washington: Government Printing Office, 1888), 200–1, 350–1.

14. Quoted in *Annual Report of the Supervising Surgeon-General of the Marine-Hospital Service of the United States for the Fiscal Year 1892* (Washington: Government Printing Office, 1893), 139. It was Dr. Gardner who later had the melancholy duty of declaring Captain Healy insane after the latter had tried several times to kill himself during the voyage of the cutter *McCulloch* in 1900. Healy had been drinking heavily for years. See Gary C. Stein, "A desperate and dangerous man: Captain Michael A. Healy's arctic cruise of 1900," *Alaska Journal* 15 (2): 39–45, Spring 1985.

15. Quoted in *Annual Report of the Supervising Surgeon-General of the Marine-Hospital Service of the United States for the Fiscal Year 1895* (Washington: Government Printing Office, 1896), 180–1.

16. Although nearly all medical officers on revenue cutters in Alaska were from the Marine-Hospital Service, Dr. Call may have been a direct hire.

17. *Annual Report of the Revenue-Marine Service, 1891* (Washington: Government Printing Office, 1891).

18. D. H. Jarvis, *Report of the Cruise of the US Revenue Cutter* Bear *and the Overland Expedition for the Relief of the Whalers in the Arctic Ocean from November 27, 1897, to September 13, 1898.* Treasury Department Document No. 2101 (Washington: Government Printing Office, 1899). Dr. Call's report, dated September 1, 1898, appears at the end of the document. See also Albert K. Cocke, "Dr. Samuel Call," *Alaska Journal* 4 (3): 181–88, Summer 1974; William L. Boyd, "Jarvis and the reindeer caper," *Arctic*: 75–82, June 1972.

19. Evans, *United States Coast Guard*, 148–9.

20. Truman R. Strobridge and Dennis L. Noble, *Alaska and the US Revenue Cutter Service, 1867–1915* (Annapolis: Naval Institute Press, 1999), 136–37.

21. James T. White, "Diary of the cruise of the *Bear*, 1889." Typescript, John W. White and James T. White Collection, Alaska and Polar Regions Department, Rasmuson Library, University of Alaska Fairbanks.

22. James T. White, Handwritten notes, John W. White and James T. White Collection, Alaska and Polar Regions Collection, Rasmuson Library, University of Alaska Fairbanks. Box II, Folder 13.

23. James T. White, "Report of the Medical Officer, US Steamer *Nunivak*." In J. C. Cantwell, *Report of the Operations of the US Revenue Steamer Nunivak on the Yukon River Station, Alaska, 1899–1901* (Washington: Government Printing Office, 1902), 257–74.

24. Gary C. Stein, "Ship's surgeon on the Yukon," *Alaska Journal, A 1981 Collection*, edited by Virginia McKinney (Anchorage: Alaska Northwest Publishing Company, 1981), 228–36.

25. John G. Brady, *Report of the Governor of the District of Alaska to the Secretary of the Interior, 1903* (Washington: Government Printing Office, 1903), 28. Brady was of course wrong that the MHS physicians were ever charging for their services.

26. Ted C. Hinckley, ed., "Dr. Friench Simpson, US Public Health Service, describes his adventures aboard the USRC *Commodore Perry*, in Alaskan waters, 1909," *Alaska Medicine* 14: 123–28, October 1972.

27. H. E. Hasseltine, "Report of Asst. Surg. H. E. Hasseltine," in "Sanitary conditions in Alaska," *Public Health Reports* 26(18): 631–36, May 5, 1911. In his later PHS career Dr. Hasseltine worked in the field of psittacosis and leprosy (PHS personnel records).

28. J. A. Watkins, "The Alaskan Eskimo: The prevalence of disease and the sanitary conditions of the villages along the arctic coast," *American Journal of Public Health* 4: 643–48, August 1914.

29. *Annual Report of the US Revenue-Cutter Service, 1914*, Treasury Department (Washington: Government Printing Office, 1914), 139–40.

30. United States Department of the Interior, Bureau of Education, "Report on the Work of the Bureau of Education for the Natives of Alaska, 1913–14," *Bureau of Education Bulletin* No. 48 (Washington: Government Printing Office, 1915), 6; *Annual Report of the Cutter Service, 1914*, 146–48; Dennis L. Noble and Truman R. Strobridge, "The Revenue Cutter *Tahoma*," *Alaska Journal* 6 (2): 118–22, Spring 1976.

31. *Annual Report of the Surgeon General of the Public Health Service of the United States for the Fiscal Year 1914* (Washington: Government Printing Office, 1914), 294–95.

32. Starting in FY1925, the dental officer assigned to the Bering Sea Patrol maintained an office at Unalaska. See *Annual Report of the Surgeon General of the Public Health Service of the United States for the Fiscal Year 1925* (Washington: Government Printing Office, 1925), 200.

33. *Annual Report of the Surgeon General of the Public Health Service of the United States for the Fiscal Year 1916* (Washington: Government Printing Office, 1916), 3436.

34. Thomas Riggs Jr., *Report of the Governor of Alaska to the Secretary of the Interior 1919* (Washington: Government Printing Office, 1919), 11; Strobridge and Noble, *Alaska and the Cutter Service*, 134–35.

35. Dennis Noble, "Fog, men, and cutters: A short history of the Bering Sea Patrol," US Coast Guard Website: http://www.uscg.mil/hq/g-cp/history/BeringSea.html (1999)

36. William Bixby, *Track of the* Bear (New York: David McKay Company, 1965), 145–46.

37. William A. Kelly to John Brady, in Brady, *Report of the Governor, 1900*, 52.

38. Thomas Parran et al. *Alaska's Health, A Survey Report* (Pittsburgh: University of Pittsburgh Graduate School of Public Health, 1954), IV-72.

39. *Annual Report of the Surgeon General of the Public Health Service of the United States for the Fiscal Year 1929* (Washington: Government Printing Office, 1929), 231.

40. George A. Parks, *Annual Report of the Governor of Alaska to the Secretary of the Interior for the Fiscal Year Ended June 30, 1932* (Washington: Government Printing Office, 1932), 22.

41. *Annual Report of the Surgeon General of the Public Health Service of the United States for the Fiscal Year 1935* (Washington: Government Printing Office, 1935), 110.

Chapter 3

1. George W. Bailey, *Report upon Alaska and Its People* (Washington: Government Printing Office, 1880), 24.

2. *Annual Report of the Supervising Surgeon-General of the Marine-Hospital Service of the United States, for the Fiscal Year 1880* (Washington: Government Printing Office, 1880), 47.

3. This was officially designated as a "Class 3 Relief Station." *Annual Report of the Supervising Surgeon-General of the Marine-Hospital Service of the United States, for the Fiscal Year 1882* (Washington: Government Printing Office, 1882), 56; *Annual Report of the Supervising Surgeon-General of the Marine-Hospital Service of the United States, for the Fiscal Year 1883* (Washington: Government Printing Office, 1883), 16.

4. Zina Pitcher, "Medicine in Alaska," *The Medical Age* 4: 510–12, 1886.

5. *Annual Report of the Supervising Surgeon-General of the Marine-Hospital Service of the United States, for the Fiscal Year 1889* (Washington: Government Printing Office, 1889), 127, 416.

6. *Annual Report of the Supervising Surgeon-General of the Marine-Hospital Service of the United States for the Fiscal Year 1897* (Washington: Government Printing Office, 1898), 45, 344–5.

7. Samuel C. Leonhardt, in Brady, *Report of the Governor of Alaska, 1900*, 61.

8. *Annual Report of the Supervising Surgeon-General of the Marine-Hospital Service of the United States for the Fiscal Year 1893* (Washington: Government Printing Office, 1894), 139.

9. Truman R. Strobridge and Dennis L. Noble, *Alaska and the US Revenue Cutter Service, 1867–1915* (Annapolis: Naval Institute Press, 1999), 134–35.

10. *Annual Report of the Supervising Surgeon-General of the Marine-Hospital Service of the United States for the Fiscal Year 1900* (Washington: Government Printing Office, n.d.), 12.

11. Dunlop Moore, "Inspection service at Dutch Harbor," *Public Health Reports* 15(31): 1928, August 3, 1900.

12. Dunlop Moore, quoted in John G. Brady, *Report of the Governor of the District of Alaska to the Secretary of the Interior, 1900* (Washington: Government Printing Office), 61.

13. Brady, *Report of the Governor, 1900*, 36.

14. Charles N. Vogel, in John G. Brady, *Report of the Governor of the District of Alaska to the Secretary of the Interior, 1902* (Washington: Government Printing Office, 1902), Appendix K, 92.

15. *Operations of the United States Public Health and Marine-Hospital Service, 1903* (Washington: Government Printing Office, n.d.), 18–19.

16. *Annual Report of the Surgeon-General of the Public Health and Marine-Hospital Service of the United States for the Fiscal Year 1905* (Washington: Government Printing Office, n.d.), 378–80.

17. Joseph Herman Romig, in John G. Brady, *Report of the Governor of the District Alaska to the Secretary of the Interior, 1905* (Washington: Government Printing Office, 1905), 32.

18. Tim Troll, "Kanakanak Hospital celebrates 90 years," *Bristol Bay Times*, December 11, 2003.

19. Strobridge and Noble, *Alaska and the US Revenue Cutter Service*, 136.

20. *Annual Report of the Surgeon-General of the Public Health and Marine-Hospital Service of the United States for the Fiscal Year 1907* (Washington: Government Printing Office, 1908), 107.

21. George A. Parks, *Report of the Governor of Alaska to the Secretary of the Interior, 1926* (Washington: Government Printing Office, 1926), 91.

22. George A. Parks, *Report of the Governor of Alaska to the Secretary of the Interior, 1928* (Washington: Government Printing Office, 1928); *Report of the Governor of Alaska to the Secretary of the Interior, 1929* (Washington: Government Printing Office, 1929), 88.

23. John Troy, *Annual Report of the Governor of Alaska to the Secretary of the Interior for the Fiscal Year Ended June 30, 1936* (Washington: Government Printing Office, 1936), 32.

24. *Annual Report of the Surgeon General of the Public Health Service of the United States for the Fiscal Year 1936* (Washington: Government Printing Office, 1936), 112.

25. Ernest Gruening, *Annual Report of the Governor of Alaska to the Secretary of the Interior for the Fiscal Year Ended June 30, 1941* (Washington: Government Printing Office, 1941), 56.

Chapter 4

1. Letter from D. H. Jarvis to the Secretary of the Treasury, June 28, 1900, quoted in *Annual Report of the Supervising Surgeon-General of the Marine-Hospital Service of the United States for the Fiscal Year 1900* (Washington: Government Printing Office, 1900), 618–19.

2. Telegram from D. H. Jarvis to the Secretary of the Treasury, June 29, 1900, quoted in *Annual Report of the Surgeon-General for the Fiscal Year 1900*, 619; Telegram from D. H. Jarvis to the Secretary of the Treasury, July 2, 1900, quoted in *Annual Report of the Surgeon-General for the Fiscal Year 1900*, 619.

3. Telegram from Walter Wyman to Bayliss Earle, July 11, 1900, quoted in *Annual Report of the Surgeon-General for the Fiscal Year 1900*, 620.

4. James T. White, "Report of the medical officer US Steamer *Nunivak*," in J. C. Cantwell, *Report of the Operations of the US Revenue Steamer* Nunivak *on the Yukon River Station, Alaska, 1899–1901* (Washington: Government Printing Office, 1902), 257–59.

5. Dunlop Moore, "Inspection service at Dutch Harbor," *Public Health Reports* 15 (31): 1928, August 3, 1900.

6. See *Public Health Reports* 15(31): 1925–28 , August 3, 1900.

7. John G. Brady, *Report of the Governor of Alaska, 1901* (Washington: Government Printing Office, 1901), 35.

8. Carroll Fox, "Report of Officer Detailed to Investigate Smallpox in Alaska," in *Annual Report of the Supervising Surgeon-General of the Marine-Hospital Service of the United States, for the Fiscal Year 1901* (Washington, Government Printing Office, n.d.), 579–82. Fox, incidentally, went on to a 37-year career with the PHS and retired as the Chief Quarantine Officer for the Port of New York (PHS personnel records).

9. J. C. Kooshner, "A Second Case of Smallpox on the U. S. Fish Commission Steamer *Albatross*, at Sitka, Alaska," *Public Health Reports* 16: 1976–77, August 30, 1901.

10. Samuel C. Leonhardt, "End of Smallpox at Juneau and Douglas City, Alaska," *Public Health Reports* 17: 1551, July 4, 1902.

11. *Annual Report of the Supervising Surgeon-General of the Marine-Hospital Service of the United States for the Fiscal Year 1901* (Washington: Government Printing Office, n.d.), 482.

12. *Annual Report of the Surgeon-General of the Public Health and Marine-Hospital Service of the United States for the Fiscal Year 1902* (Washington: Government Printing Office, n.d.), 280.

13. Samuel C. Leonhardt, "A Case of Smallpox from Juneau, Alaska," *Public Health Reports* 17: 1551, July 4, 1902; *Annual Report of the Surgeon-General for FY1902*, 411.

14. *Annual Report of the Surgeon General of the Public Health and Marine-Hospital Service of the United States for the Fiscal Year 1911* (Washington: Government Printing Office, n.d.), 139–40, 230–1.

15. *Annual Report of the Surgeon General of the Public Health Service of the United States for the Fiscal Year 1912* (Washington: Government Printing Office, 1913), 175.

16. *Annual Report of the Surgeon General of the Public Health Service of the United States for the Fiscal Year 1914* (Washington: Government Printing Office, 1914), 249.

17. *Public Health Reports*, May 12, 1916, 1208.

18. Ronald L. Lautaret, "Alaska's greatest disaster: The 1918 Spanish influenza epidemic," *Alaska Journal 1986*, edited by Terrence Cole, 16: 238–43, 1986.

19. "The Work of the Bureau of Education for the Natives of Alaska," from the *Biennial Survey of Education in the United States, 1918–1920*, US Department of the Interior, Bureau of Education (Washington: Government Printing Office, 1921), 9.

20. George A. Parks, *Report of the Governor of Alaska to the Secretary of the Interior, 1926* (Washington: Government Printing Office, 1926), 89–90.

21. George A. Parks, *Report of the Governor of Alaska to the Secretary of the Interior, 1925* (Washington: Government Printing Office, 1925), 76.

22. *Annual Report of the Surgeon General of the Public Health Service of the United States for the Fiscal Year 1925* (Washington: Government Printing Office, 1925), 222.

23. Gay Salisbury and Laney Salisbury, *The Cruelest Miles: The Heroic Story of Dogs and Men in a Race Against an Epidemic* (New York: W.W. Norton & Co., 2003), 51; George A. Parks, *Report of the Governor of Alaska to the Secretary of the Interior, 1925* (Washington: Government Printing Office, 1925), 75.

24. William H. Wilson, "The serum dash to Nome, 1925: The making of Alaskan heroes," *Alaska Journal* 16: 250–59, 1986.

25. *Annual Report of the Surgeon General of the Public Health Service of the United States for the Fiscal Year 1927* (Washington: Government Printing Office, 1927), 249.

26. L. L. Lumsden, "Illness among Chinese recently returned from salmon canneries of Alaska," *Public Health Reports* 15: 2795–98, November 16, 1900.

27. D. H. Currie, "Beriberi, or a disease closely resembling it, met in Chinese returning to San Francisco from Alaska," *American Medicine* 6: 225–27, 1903.

28. Parks, *Report of the Governor of Alaska, 1926*, 90–91.

29. *Annual Report of the Surgeon General for FY1927*, 312.

30. *Annual Report of the Surgeon General of the Public Health Service of the United States for the Fiscal Year 1931* (Washington: Government Printing Office, 1931), 141, 157; *Annual Report of the Surgeon General of the Public Health Service of the United States for the Fiscal Year 1932* (Washington: Government Printing Office, 1932), 103.

31. *Annual Report of the Surgeon General of the Public Health Service of the United States for the Fiscal Year 1935* (Washington: Government Printing Office, 1935), 74; *Annual Report of the Surgeon General of the Public Health Service of the United States for the Fiscal Year 1939* (Washington: Government Printing Office, 1939), 94.

32. George A. Parks, *Annual Report of the Governor of Alaska to the Secretary of the Interior, 1931* (Washington: Government Printing Office, 1931), 116; John W. Troy, *Annual Report of the Governor of Alaska to the Secretary of the*

Interior, for the Fiscal Year Ended June 30, 1934 (Washington: Government Printing Office, 1934), 35.

33. Public Law 271, 74th Cong. [H.R. 7260], approved Aug. 14, 1935.

34. *Second Annual Report, Federal Security Agency, 1941* (Washington: Government Printing Office, 1941), 104.

35. *Annual Report of the Surgeon General for the Fiscal Year 1939*, 137, 142.

Chapter 5

1. Ralph Chester Williams, *The United States Public Health Service, 1798–1950* (Washington: Commissioned Officers Association of the USPHS, 1950), 735–37.

2. Ernest Gruening, *Annual Report of the Governor of Alaska to the Secretary of the Interior for the Fiscal Year Ended June 30, 1944* (Washington: Government Printing Office, 1944), 18–19.

3. Carl E. Buck and George A. Hays, "Public health needs in Alaska," *Alaska's Health* 1 (1): June 1943.

4. Ernest Gruening, *Annual Report of the Governor of Alaska to the Secretary of the Interior for the Fiscal Year Ended June 30, 1945* (Washington: Government Printing Office, 1945), 18.

5. *Annual Report of the Federal Security Agency, Section Four, United States Public Health Service, for the Fiscal Year 1945* (Washington: Government Printing Office, 1945), 280.

6. *Annual Report of the Federal Security Agency for the Fiscal Year 1946* (Washington: Government Printing Office, 1946), 370–1.

7. "Dr. Gehrig joins staff," *Alaska's Health* 4 (4): April 1946.

8. *Annual Report of the Federal Security Agency, Section Three, United States Public Health Service, for the Fiscal Year 1947* (Washington: Government Printing Office, 1947), 462.

9. Ernest Gruening, "Arctic Health Institute in Alaska," Memo to the Bureau of the Budget, April 27, 1949.

10. Christine A. Heller, Alaska Nutrition Survey Report (Juneau: Territorial Department of Health, 1947).

11. Joseph D. Aronson, "BCG vaccination among American Indians," *American Review of Tuberculosis* 57 (1): 96–99, January 1948; T. H. Rose, "Alaska's hospital needs," *Alaska's Health* 5: December 1947; "Albrecht's trip profitable," *Alaska's Health* 6 (2): February 1948.

12. *Annual Report of the Federal Security Agency, 1949, Public Health Service* (Washington: Government Printing Office, 1949), 143–45.

13. C. Earl Albrecht, "The Alaska Health Plan," *Alaska's Health* 6 (7–8): July-August 1948; "Around Alaska," *Alaska's Health* 6 (9): September 1948; "Latest TB report shows 5,279 cases in Alaska; brings ratio to 1 in 20," *Alaska's Health* 8 (3–4): March–April 1950.

14. "Alaska's tuberculosis vaccination work is resumed," *Alaska's Health* 9: June 1952; "Health ships tied up as result of fund slashes: Many remote areas lose sole medical aid as three marine units cease work," *Alaska's Health* 9: October 1952.

15. Press Release, Alaska Department of Health, Juneau, Alaska, May 31, 1955.

16. The first active-duty Surgeon General of the Public Health Service to come to Alaska was Luther Terry, who visited in the summer of 1964. On a wide-ranging tour he inspected earthquake damage at the PHS Alaska Native Hospital in Anchorage, dedicated the new Arctic Health Research Center building at the University of Alaska in Fairbanks, and even paid a visit to Barrow. The next to fly north was Surgeon General William Stewart, who visited Alaska in the summer of 1967.

17. Thomas Parran et al., *Alaska's Health: A Survey Report* (Pittsburgh: University of Pittsburgh Graduate School of Public Health, 1954).

18. Keith R. Hooker, "A new approach to tuberculosis in Alaska," *NTRDA Bulletin*, July–August 1968: 9–12.

19. Department of Health, Education and Welfare, Public Health Service, "Report of Alaska Mental Health Survey," Typescript (1956); *Annual Report, US Department of Health, Education, and Welfare, 1957* (Washington: Government Printing Office, 1957), 132.

20. *HEW 1959: Annual Report of the US Department of Health, Education, and Welfare* (Washington: Government Printing Office, 1959), 118.

21. Dr. Eisenberg later went on to become a distinguished clinician, teacher, and author at the University of Washington School of Medicine.

22. John Middaugh, Personal communication, July 27, 2004.

Chapter 6

1. *Annual Report of the Supervising Surgeon-General of the Marine-Hospital Service of the United States for the Fiscal Year 1883* (Washington: Government Printing Office, 1883), 16–18.

2. John G. Brady, *Report of the Governor of Alaska, 1901* (Washington: Government Printing Office, 1901), 50.

3. Carroll Fox, "Tuberculosis among the Indians of Southeast Alaska," *Public Health Reports* 16: 1615–16, 1902.

4. Brady, *Report of the Governor of Alaska, 1901*, 50.

5. *Annual Report of the Surgeon General of the Public Health and Marine-Hospital Service of the United States for the Fiscal Year 1911* (Washington: Government Printing Office, 1911), 229.

6. *Annual Report of the Surgeon General for FY 1911*, 229–30.

7. Milton H. Foster, "Reports of Dr. Milton H. Foster," in *Report on Education of the Natives of Alaska and the Reindeer Service, 1910–11*, US Bureau of Education, Alaska School Service, Whole No. 484 (Washington: Government Printing Office, 1912), 66–76.

8. Foster, "Reports" (1912): 76.

9. Letter from Emil Krulish to the Surgeon General, July 26, 1915, PHS personnel records.

10. Emil Krulish and Daniel S. Neuman, *Medical Handbook*, Department of the Interior, Bureau of Education: Alaska School Service (Washington: Government Printing Office, 1913).

11. See Emil Krulish, "Sanitary conditions in Alaska," *Public Health Reports* 28: 544–51, March 21, 1913; "Sanitary conditions among the Eskimos: A report on conditions in native villages along the arctic coast of Alaska," *Public Health Reports*, Supplement No. 9, December 12, 1913; "Sanitary conditions in Alaska: A report upon the diseases found among the Indians of southeastern Alaska," *Public Health Reports* 29: 1300–4, May 22, 1914. Additional reports by Krulish were published in the *Annual Reports of the Bureau of Education*.

12. Emil Krulish, "Teaching health to the Eskimo: United States government work in Alaska," *Mother and Child* 2: 151–58, 1921.

13. *Annual Report of the Surgeon General of the Public Health Service of the United States for the Fiscal Year 1914* (Washington: Government Printing Office, 1914), 248.

14. *Annual Report of the Surgeon General of the Public Health Service of the United States for the Fiscal Year 1915* (Washington: Government Printing Office, 1915), 264.

15. *Annual Report of the Surgeon General of the Public Health Service of the United States for the Fiscal Year 1916* (Washington: Government Printing Office, 1916), 272.

16. Letter from Emil Krulish to Governor Thomas Riggs Jr., April 13, 1919. NARA RG 80-14, Roll 63. The governor and the surgeon general continued to correspond on the subject, and on December 18 Blue wrote to the Assistant Secretary of the Interior that he was unable to help the governor because "The Service itself is terribly handicapped for the want of competent medical men," as a result of its expanded service to the care of "ex-soldiers of the late war." Ultimately, a local Juneau practitioner took on the job part time. *See* Letter from Thomas Riggs Jr. to Rupert Blue, June 17, 1919, NARA RG80-14, Roll 58; Letter from Rupert Blue to John W. Hallowell, December 18, 1919, NARA RG80-14, Roll 63.

17. PHS personnel records.

18. US Department of the Interior, *Annual Report of the Commissioner of Indian Affairs to the Secretary of the Interior for the Fiscal Year ended June 30, 1932* (Washington: Government Printing Office, 1932), 12.

19. F. S. Fellows, "Mortality in the native races of the Territory of Alaska, with special reference to tuberculosis," *Public Health Reports* 49(9): 289–98, March 2, 1934. After leaving Alaska, Fellows spent one more year with Indian health in New Mexico. During World War II he saw combat with the Coast Guard (PHS personnel records).

20. United States Department of the Interior, *Annual Report of the Secretary of the Interior for the Fiscal Year Ended June 30, 1935* (Washington: Government Printing Office, 1935), 139.

21. J. F. Van Ackeren, "Statement of Dr. J. F. Van Ackern [sic], Medical Director, Indian Service for Alaska, August 17, 1936," United States Congress, Senate Committee on Indian Affairs, *Survey of Conditions on the Indians in the United States*, Part 36: Alaska, including Reindeer, 74th Congress, 2nd Session (Washington: Government Printing Office, 1939), 19865–70.

22. United States Department of the Interior, *Annual Report of the Secretary of the Interior for the Fiscal Year Ending June 30, 1937* (Washington: Government Printing Office, 1937), 238.

23. Letter from Edgar W. Norris to Rudolph Haas, February 5, 1945, NARA RG80-14, R248; Rudolf Haas, "A tuberculosis control program for Alaska," *Alaska's Health* 4 (4): April 1945.

24. Margaret Cantwell and Mary George Edmond, *North to Share: The Sisters of Saint Ann in Alaska and the Yukon Territory* (Victoria, B.C.: Sisters of St. Ann, 1992), 187–91.

25. *Annual Report of the Federal Security Agency, Section Four, United States Public Health Service, for the Fiscal Year 1945* (Washington: Government Printing Office, 1945), 274–75.

26. PHS personnel records.

27. Harry Barnett, Jack Fields, George Milles, Joseph Silverstein, and Arthur Bernstein, "Medical conditions in Alaska: A report by a group sent by the American Medical Association," *Journal of the American Medical Association* 135 (8): 500–10, 1947.

28. Frank H. Douglass, David B. Law, W. Charles Martin, Austin T. Moore, John E. Tuhy, "Medical conditions in Alaska: A progress report," Unpublished typescript, October 29, 1948.

29. Kenneth Kastella, Interview with Philip Moore at Sequim, Washington, Typescript, no date.

30. "Vaccinations against TB given to 2,486 Alaskans in past year; BCG vaccine given in 41 Kenai-to-Barrow villages," *Alaska's Health* 10: June 1953.

31. Robert Fortuine, "E. S. ('Stu') Rabeau, 1920–1984," *Alaska Medicine* 26(3): 95–96, 1984.

Chapter 7

1. Ruth M. Raup, "The Indian health program from 1800–1955," US Department of Health Education and Welfare, Public Health Service (March 11, 1959).

2. "US Public Health Service Alaska Information," Pamphlet, USPHS/Bureau of Medical Services/Alaska Native Health Service, n.d., 1–2.

3. *Annual Report, US Department of Health, Education, and Welfare, 1956* (Washington: Government Printing Office, 1956), 120–25; *Annual Report, US Department of Health, Education and Welfare, 1957* (Washington: Government Printing Office, 1957), 120.

4. An old Alaskan saying from the Russian era went thus: "God is in heaven and the Czar is in St. Petersburg."

5. In 1963 Kasuga went on to Washington and later served as Deputy Director of the Division of Indian Health and Associate Director of the Bureau of Medical Services at the grade of Assistant Surgeon General (PHS Personnel records). He died in 2003.

6. This second group is of special interest, since many, following their draft commitment, set up private practice in Alaska, thus greatly strengthening the profession in the state. It is also notable that four former PHS commissioned officers from the IHS have become directors of the State Division of Public Health, including E. S. Rabeau, Robert Fraser, Peter Nakamura, and Richard Mandsager.

7. A few articles by PHS physicians in the field hospitals give the range of their experiences: Harriet Jackson, "Tundra practice, present and future," *Alaska Medicine* 1: 118–19, December 1959; "Don Schultz, '50, wilderness medic," *Ursina College Bulletin* (March 1959); Dudley J. Weider, "A physician visits Little Diomede," *HSMHA Health Reports* 86 (1): 9–16, January 1971; Dudley J. Weider, "Arctic doctor," *HSMHA World*:16–20, Nov/Dec 1968.

8. Dr. Edwards published a case report on brucellosis in the Arctic in an early issue of *Alaska Medicine*. Stan Edwards, "*Brucella suis* in the Arctic," *Alaska Medicine* 1 (2): 41-44, June 1959.

9. Robert Fortuine, *Alaska Native Medical Center: A History, 1953–1983* (Anchorage: Alaska Native Medical Center, Alaska Area Native Health Service, 1986), 146–47.

10. Dr. Wherritt became Chief, Office of Program Services, at IHS headquarters, then went on to the grade of Assistant Surgeon General as Director of the PHS District at Kansas City, Missouri. He died in 2002.

11. *HEW 1959: Annual Report of the US Department of Health, Education and Welfare* (Washington: Government Printing Office, 1959), 142.

12. *Annual Report, 1965, US Department of Health, Education and Welfare* (Washington: Government Printing Office, 1965), 156.

13. "Eskimos, Indians and Aleuts of Alaska: A Digest, Anchorage Area" (Washington: US Department of Health, Education and Welfare, PHS, BMS, DIH, March 1963), 12.

14. *Annual Report, US Department of Health, Education and Welfare, 1960* (Washington: Government Printing Office, 1960), 132, 135; *Annual Report, US Department of Health, Education and Welfare, 1961* (Washington: Government Printing Office, 1961), 199.

15. *HEW 1959: Annual Report of the US Department of Health, Education and Welfare* (Washington: Government Printing Office, 1959), 107.

16. James Crum, Personal communication, October 29, 2004. Captain Crum began his PHS career in Alaska in 1967 and retired in 1996 as Director, Office of Environmental Health and Engineering, for the Alaska Area. See also "Eskimos, Indians and Aleuts of Alaska: A Digest," 11.

17. "Eskimos, Indians and Aleuts of Alaska: A Digest," 9–10.

18. Martha Richardson Wilson, "Effect of the Alaska earthquake on functions of PHS Hospital," *Public Health Reports* 79 (10): 853–61, October 1964.

19. Thomas J. Harrison, "Training for village health aides in the Kotzebue area of Alaska," *Public Health Reports* 80 (7): 565–72, July 1965; Philip Nice and Walter Johnson, *The Alaska Health Aide Program: A Tradition of Helping Ourselves* (Privately Printed, 1998).

20. Upon his retirement from the PHS in December 1975, Lee was replaced by Gerald H. Ivey, the first in a succession of Alaska Natives to hold the position up to the present time.

21. Dr. Lee retired in Alaska, where he remained active in clinical medicine and public health. He died in 1998.

22. "Description of the Program, Alaska Area Native Health Service," US Department of Health, Education and Welfare, Public Health Service,

Health Services Administration, Indian Health Service, Alaska Area Native Health Service, July 1979.

23. Heather E. Hudson and Edward B. Parker, "Medical communication in Alaska by satellite," *New England Journal of Medicine* 289: 1351–56, December 20, 1973. *See also* John B. Muth, "Martha L. Wilson, M.D.," *Alaska Medicine* 22 (3): 43–44, May/June 1980.

24. Arthur C. Willman, Personal communication, November 9, 2004. Mr. Willman died in 2005.

Chapter 8

1. US Public Health Service, "Alaska Health and Sanitation Activities: A Progress Report on Public Health in Alaska," Typescript, December 1, 1948; *Annual Report of the Federal Security Agency, 1949, Public Health Service*, 62–63.

2. Marcia Hayes, "Some problems of health in Alaska," *Proceedings of the 6th Pacific Science Conference* (1942), 465–72; C. Earl Albrecht, "A New Year's Message," *Alaska's Health* 5 (1): January 1947.

3. Harry Barnett, Jack Fields, George Milles, Joseph Silverstein, and Arthur Bernstein, "Medical conditions in Alaska: A report by a group sent by the American Medical Association," *Journal of the American Medical Association* 135 (8): 500–10, 1947.

4. C. Earl Albrecht, "The Alaska Health Plan," *Alaska's Health* 6 (7–8): July–August 1948; A. B. Colyar, "Arctic Health Research Center, an introduction," *Alaska Medicine* 1 (1): 31–33, March 1959.

5. Jack C. Haldeman, "Facilities and opportunities for research at the Arctic Health Research Center," *Public Health Reports* 66 (29): 31–34, 1951.

6. This library became the nucleus of the ANMC hospital library in the 1970s and later the foundation of the Alaska Health Sciences Library, now part of the Consortium Library of the University of Alaska Anchorage, and providing services to all of the health professions of Alaska. See M. Walter Johnson, "Alaska Health Sciences Library: A tribute, a welcome, and a challenge," *Alaska Medicine* 19 (1): 4–6, January 1977.

7. Haldeman, "Facilities and Opportunities for Research," 1951. Dr. Haldeman spent 22 years in the PHS. After leaving Alaska he served as Chief of the Division of State Grants and later as Chief of the Division of General Health Services. After July 1958 he was Chief of the Division of Hospitals and Medical Facilities, which administered the national Hill-Burton hospital construction program. He retired in 1963 as Assistant Surgeon General and died in 1985 (PHS personnel records).

8. Ernest Gruening, "Arctic Health Institute in Alaska," Memo to the Bureau of the Budget (April 27, 1949).

9. Colyar, "Arctic Health Research Center: An Introduction," 31–33.

10. "Hope Is Pinned on Congress for Approval of Appropriation for Erection of Arctic Institute of Health at Alaska University," *Alaska's Health* 8 (3–4): March–April 1950.

11. *ATA News* 6 (1): May 1953.

12. "Arctic Health Research Center Publications, 1949–1968" (College, AK: PHS/AHRC, 1968).

Appendix

Selected References Illustrating
PHS Research in Alaska

1. Arctic Health Research Center (1948–1973)

Environmental Health

Anderegg, James C., G. L. Hubbs, and E. R. Eaton. "Ice water on tap for the Arctic: Pneumatic purging system, protected by simple air-lock device, makes fill and draw water supply workable in sub-zero weather." *Water Works Engineering* 13 (7): 632–35, 1960.

Benson, Barrett E. "Treatment for high iron content in remote Alaskan water supplies." *Journal of the American Water Works Association* 58 (10): 1356–62, 1966.

Cohen, Jules B., and Barrett E. Benson. "Arctic water storage." *Journal of the American Water Works Association* 60 (3): 291–97, 1968.

Day, Elroy K. "Public health problems in Alaska: Sewage and waste disposal problems." *Public Health Reports* 66 (29): 922–28, 1951.

Duncan, David L. "Individual household recirculating waste disposal system for rural Alaska." *Journal of Water Pollution Control Federation* 36 (12): 1468–78, 1964.

Hickey, John S., Dennis R. Wik, William B. Page, and M. L. Shank. *Studies on Housing for Alaska Natives*. US Public Health Service Publication No 999-AH-l. Washington: Government Printing Office, October 1965. 127 pp.

Page, William B. "Design of Water Distribution Systems for Service in Arctic Regions." *Water and Sewage Works* 101 (8): 333–37, 1954.

Human Physiology

Anderson, Kristian Lange, A. Boistad, Y. Løyning, and L. Irving. "Physical fitness of arctic Indians." *Journal of Applied Physiology* 15 (4): 645–48, 1960.

Hildes, John A., L. Irving, and J. S. Hart. "Estimation of heat flow from hands of Eskimos by calorimetry." *Journal of Applied Physiology* 16 (4): 617–23, 1961.

Hock, Raymond J., H. Erickson, W. Flagg, P. Scholander, and L. Irving. "Composition of the ground-level atmosphere at Point Barrow." *Journal of Meteorology* 9 (6): 441–42, 1952.

Irving, L. "Public health problems in Alaska: Climatic adaptation in arctic and tropic animals." *Public Health Reports* 66: 939–41, 1951.

_____. "Human adaptation to cold." *Nature* 185 (4713): 572–74, 1960.

_____. "Effect of temperature on sensitivity of the finger." *Journal of Applied Physiology* 15 (6): 1201–5, 1963.

Irving, L., K. L. Anderson, Y. Løyning, J. D. Nelms, L. J. Peyton, and R. D. Whaley. "Metabolism and temperature of arctic Indian men during a cold night." *Journal of Applied Physiology* 15 (4): 635–44, 1960.

Miller, L. Keith, and L. Irving. "Local reactions to air cooling in an Eskimo population." *Journal of Applied Physiology* 17 (3): 449–55, 1962.

Petajan, Jack H. "Pathophysiological aspects of human adjustment to cold." *Archives of Environmental Health* 17: 595–98, 1968.

Zoonotic Diseases

Brandly, P. J., and R. L. Rausch. "A preliminary note on trichinosis investigations in Alaska." *Arctic* 3 (2): 105–6, 1950.

Fay, Francis, II, and F. S. L. Williamson. "Studies on the helminth fauna of Alaska, XXXIX: *Echinococcus multilocularis* Leuckart, 1863, and other helminths of foxes on the Pribilof Islands." *Canadian Journal of Zoology* 40: 767–72, 1962.

Rausch, Robert L. "Hydatid disease (echinococcosis) in Alaska and the importance of rodent intermediate hosts." *Science* 113 (2925): 57–58, 1951.

_____. "Public health problems in Alaska: Biotic interrelationships of helminth parasitism." *Public Health Reports* 66 (29): 928–34, 1951.

_____. "Hydatid disease in boreal regions." *Arctic* 5 (3): 157–74, 1952.

_____. "Studies on the helminth fauna of Alaska, XXX: The occurrence of *Echinococcus multilocularis* Leuckart, 1863, on the mainland of Alaska." *American Journal of Tropical Medicine and Hygiene* 5 (6): 1086–92, 1956.

_____. "Some observations on rabies in Alaska, with special reference to wild Canidae." *Journal of Wildlife Management* 22 (3): 246–60, 1958.

_____. "On the ecology and distribution of Echinococcus spp. (Cestoda: Taeniidae), and characteristics of their development in the intermediate host." *Annales de Parasitologie* (Paris) 42 (1): 19–63, 1967.

_____. "Zoonotic diseases in the changing Arctic." *Archives of Environmental Health* 17: 627–30, 1968.

Rausch, Robert L., B. B. Babero, V. R. Rausch, and H. L. Schiller. "Studies on the helminth fauna of Alaska, XXVII: The occurrence of larvae of *Trichinella spiralis* in Alaskan mammals." *Journal of Parasitology* 42 (3): 259–71, 1956.

Rausch, Robert L., and E. L. Schiller, "Studies on the helminth fauna of Alaska, XXXV: *Echinococcus sibiricensis* n.sp. from St. Lawrence Island." *Journal of Parasitology* 40 (6): 659–62, 1954.

_____. "Studies on the helminth fauna of Alaska, XXV: The ecology and public health significance of *Echinococcus sibiricensis* Rausch and

Schiller, 1954, on St. Lawrence Island. *Journal of Parasitology* 46 (3–4): 395–419, 1956.

Rausch, Robert L., E. M. Scott, and V. R. Rausch, "Helminths in Eskimos in western Alaska, with particular reference to *Diphyllobothrium* infection and anaemia." *Transactions of the Royal Society of Tropical Medicine and Hygiene* 61 (3): 351–57, 1967.

Wilson, Joseph F., Albert C. Diddams, and Robert L. Rausch. "Cystic hydatid disease in Alaska." *American Review of Respiratory Disease* 98 (1): 1–15, 1968.

Entomology

Berg, Clifford O. "A preliminary survey of the biting diptera of the lower Yukon Valley." In *Science in Alaska*. Proc., 2nd Alaskan Sci. Conf., Alaska Div., AAAS (1951): 303–8.

Frohne, William C. "Seasonal incidence of mosquitoes in the Upper Cook Inlet, Alaska." *Mosquito News* 11 (14): 213–16, 1951.

_____. "Biology of an Alaskan mosquito, *Culiseta alaskanensis* (Ludi.). *Annals of the Entomological Society of America* 47 (1): 9–24, 1954.

_____. "Mosquito distribution in Alaska with especial reference to a new type of life cycle." *Mosquito News* 14 (1): 10–13, 1954.

_____. "The Biology of Northern Mosquitoes." *Public Health Reports* 71, 6 (1956): 616–21, 1956.

_____. "The egg and identity of Alaskan anopheles." *Mosquito News* 16 (4): 308, 1956.

Frohne, William C., and D. A. Sleeper. "Reconnaissance of mosquitoes, punkies, and black flies in Southeast Alaska." *Mosquito News* 11 (4): 209–13, 1951.

Gjullin, C. M., D. A. Sleeper and C. N. Husman. "Control of black fly larvae in Alaskan Streams by aerial application of DDT." *Journal of Economic Entomology* 42 (2): 392, 1949.

Sommerman, Kathryn M. "True-false key to species of Alaskan biting mosquitoes." *Mosquito News* 26 (4): 540–43, 1966.

US Public Health Service, Arctic Health Research Center. "Alaskan biting flies and their control." Anchorage, 1960. 4 pp.

Wilson, Charles S. "Aerosol spray units for control of biting insects." *Mosquito News* 10 (2): 51–54, 1950.

_____. "Public health problems in Alaska: Control of Alaskan biting insects." *Public Health Reports* 66 (29): 917–22, 1951.

Nutrition and Biochemistry

Heller, Christine A., and Edward M. Scott. *The Alaska Dietary Survey 1956–61*. US Public Health Service Publication No. 999-AH-2, Environmental Health Series-Arctic Health. Washington: Government Printing Office, 1967.

Gutsche, Brett, E. M. Scott, and R. C. Wright. "Hereditary deficiency of pseudocholinesterase in Eskimos." *Nature* 215 (98): 322–23, July 15,

1967.

Petajan, J. H., G. L. Momberger, J. Aase, and D. G. Wright. "Arthrogryposis syndrome (Kuskokwim Disease) in the Eskimo." *Journal of the American Medical Association* 209 (10): 1481–86, September 8, 1969.

Scott, E. M., and D. D. Hoskins. "Hereditary methemoglobinemia in Alaskan Eskimos and Indians." *Blood* 13 (8): 795–802, 1958.

Scott, E. M., D. D. Weaver, R. C. Wright. "Discrimination of phenotypes in human serum cholinesterase deficiency." *American Journal of Human Genetics* 22: 363–69, July 1970.

Scott, E. M., and R. F. Powers. "Human serum cholinesterase, a tetramer." *Nature. New Biology* 236: 83–84, March 22, 1972.

Scott, E. M., R. C. Wright, and D. D. Weaver. "The discrimination of phenotypes for rate of disappearance of isonicotinoyl hydrazide from serum." *Journal of Clinical Investigation* 481: 1173–76, July 1969.

Epidemiology

Bender, T. R., T. S. Jones, W. E. DeWitt, et al. "Salmonellosis associated with whale meat in an Eskimo community: Serologic and bacteriologic methods as adjuncts to an epidemiologic investigation." *American Journal of Epidemiology* 96: 153–60, August 1972.

Bender, T. R., R. A. Zimmerman, J. D. Knostman, et al. "Streptococcal surveillance in remote arctic populations the development of a system for detection of group A pharyngitis and the prevention of nonsuppurative sequelae. *Acta Socio-Medica Scandinavica*, Suppl 6: 240–8, 1972.

Boyd, David, J. E. Maynard, and L. H. Hammes. "Accident mortality in Alaska, 1958–62." *Archives of Environmental Health* 17: 101–6, 1968.

Brody, Jacob A. "The infectiousness of rubella and the possibility of reinfection." *American Journal of Public Health* 56 (7): 1082–87, 1966.

Brody, Jacob A., E. R. Alexander, and M. L. Hanson. "Measles vaccine field trials in Alaska, III: Two-year follow-up of inactivated vaccine followed by live attenuated vaccine and of immune globulin with live, attenuated vaccine." *Journal of the American Medical Association* 196 (9): 757–60, 1966.

Brody, Jacob A., and E. Bridenbaugh. "Prophylactic gamma-globulin and live measles vaccine in an island epidemic of measles." *Lancet* 11: 811–13, 1964.

Brody, Jacob A., and R. Haseley. "A measles epidemic in an Alaskan boarding school." *Northwest Medicine* 54: 938–41, 1965.

Brody, Jacob A., R. McAlister, I. Emanuel, and E. R. Alexander. "Measles vaccine field trials in Alaska, I: Killed vaccine followed by live attenuated vaccine and gamma-globulin with live attenuated vaccine." *Journal of the American Medical Association* 189: 339–42, 1964.

_____. "Measles vaccine field trials in Alaska, II: Vaccination on St. Paul Island, Pribilofs, where measles had been absent for 21 years." *Journal of the American Medical Association* 190: 966–86, 1964.

Brody, Jacob A., T. Overfield, and L. M. Hammes, "Depression of the tuberculin reaction by viral vaccines." *New England Journal of Medicine* 271: 1294–96, 1964.

Brody, Jacob A., T. Overfield, and R. McAlister. "Draining ears and deafness among Alaskan Eskimos." *Archives of Otolaryngology* 81: 29–33, 1965.

Brody, Jacob A., J. L. Sever, R. McAlister, et al. "Rubella epidemic on St. Paul Island in the Pribilofs, I: Epidemiologic, clinical, and serologic findings." *Journal of the American Medical Association* 191: 619–23, 1963.

Clark, P. S., K. M. Brownsberger, A. R. Saslow, et al. "Bear meat trichinosis: Epidemiologic, serologic, and clinical observations from two Alaskan outbreaks." *Annals of Internal Medicine* 76: 951–6, June 1972.

Clark, P. S., Elmer T. Feltz, B. List-Young, et al. "An influenza B epidemic within a remote Alaska community: Serologic, epidemiologic and clinical observations." *Journal of the American Medical Association* 214: 507–12, October 19, 1970.

Duncan, I. W., and E. M. Scott. "Lactose intolerance in Alaskan Indians and Eskimos." *American Journal of Clinical Nutrition* 25: 867–8, September 1972.

Feltz, E. T., B. List-Young, D. G. Ritter, et al. "California encephalitis virus: Serological evidence of human infections in Alaska." *Canadian Journal of Microbiology* 18: 757–62, 1972.

Kaplan, G. J., P. S. Clark, T. R. Bender, et al. "Echovirus type 30 meningitis and related febrile illness: Epidemiologic study of an outbreak in an Eskimo community." *American Journal of Epidemiology* 92: 257–65, October 1970.

Fournelle, Harold J. "A seasonal study of enteric infections in Alaskan Eskimos." *Public Health Reports* 74 (1): 55–59, 1959.

Fournelle, Harold J., I. L. Wallace, and V. Radar. "A bacteriological and parasitological survey of enteric infections in an Alaskan Eskimo area." *American Journal of Public Health* 48 (11): 1489–97, 1958.

Hammes, Laurie M. "Characteristics of housing for the Yukon-Kuskokwim Delta of Southwestern Alaska." *Alaska Medicine* 7 (1): 7–10, 1965.

Maynard, James E., H. B. Dull, M. L. Hanson, E. T. Feltz, R. Berger, and L. Hammes. "Evaluation of monovalent and polyvalent influenza vaccines during an epidemic of type A2 and B influenza." *American Journal of Epidemiology* 87 (1): 148–57, 1968.

Maynard, J. E., J. K. Fleshman, and C. F. Tschopp. "Otitis media in Alaskan Eskimo children: Prospective evaluation of chemoprophylaxis." *Journal of the American Medical Association* 219: 597–99, January 31, 1972.

Maynard, J. E., and L. M. Hammes. "A study of growth, morbidity and mortality among Eskimo infants of Western Alaska." *Bulletin of the World Health Organization* 42: 613–22, 1970.

Maynard, James E., L. N. Hammes, and F. E. Kester. "Mortality due to heart disease among Alaskan Natives." *Public Health Reports* 82 (8): 714–20, 1967.

Maynard, James E., and F. P. Pauls. "Trichinosis in Alaska: A review and report of two out-breaks due to bear meat with observations on sero-diagnosis and skin testing." *American Journal of Hygiene* 76 (3): 252–61, 1962.

McAlister, Robert, J. A. Brody, and T. M. Overfield. "Enteric disease due to enteropathogenic *Escherichia coli* in hospitalized infants in Kotzebue, Alaska." *Journal of Pediatrics* 66 (2): 343–48, 1965.

Philip, Robert N., and D. Lackman. "Observations on the present distribution of influenza A/Swine antibodies among Alaskan Natives Relative to the occurrence of influenza in 1918–1919." *American Journal of Hygiene* 75 (3): 322–34, 1962.

Philip, Robert N., and K. Reinhard. "Mumps epidemic on St. Lawrence Island." In *Science in Alaska*, Proc., 8th Alaskan Sci. Conf., Alaska Div., AAAS (1957): 148–49.

Philip, Robert N., W. T. Weeks, K. R. Reinhard, D. B. Lackman, and C. French. "Observations on Asian influenza on two Alaskan islands." *Public Health Reports* 74 (8): 737–45, 1959.

Reed, D., and W. Dunn. "Epidemiologic studies of otitis media among Eskimo children." *Public Health Reports* 85: 699–706, August 1970.

Reed, Dwayne, S. Struve, and J. E. Maynard. "Otitis media and hearing deficiency among Eskimo children: A cohort study." *American Journal of Public Health* 57 (9): 1657–62, 1967.

Wulff, H., G. R. Noble, J. E. Maynard, et al. "An outbreak of respiratory infection in children associated with rhinovirus types 16 and 29." *American Journal of Epidemiology* 90: 304–11, October 1969.

Zimmerman, R. N., T. R. Bender, J. S. Edelen, and J. D. Knostman. "Streptococcal surveillance and control in Alaska Natives." *Excerpta Medica* (Amsterdam) 317: 189–97, 1972.

Tuberculosis Studies

Comstock, George W., C. Baum, and Dixie E. Snider, Jr. "Isoniazid prophylaxis among Alaskan Eskimos: A final report on the Bethel isoniazid studies." *American Review of Respiratory Disease* 119 (5): 827–29, May 1979.

Comstock, George W., and Shirley Ferebee Woolpert. "Preventive treatment of untreated, nonactive tuberculosis in an Eskimo population." *Archives of Environmental Health* 25 (5): 333–37, November 1972.

Comstock, George W., Shirley H. Ferebee, and Laurel M. Hammes. "A controlled trial of community-wide isoniazid prophylaxis in Alaska," *American Review of Respiratory Disease* 95 (6): 935–43, June 1967.

Hanson, Mary L., G. W. Comstock, and C. E. Haley. "Community isoniazid prophylaxis program in an underdeveloped area of Alaska." *Public Health Reports* 82 (12): 1045–56, December 1967.

Lear, Louise. "Chemotherapy in Alaska." *American Journal of Nursing* 57: 320–22, March 1957.

Philip, Robert N., George W. Comstock, and Joseph H. Shelton. "Phlyctenular keratoconjunctivitis among Eskimos in Southwestern Alaska, I: Epidemiologic considerations. *American Review of Respiratory Disease* 91 (2): 171–87, February 1965.

Philip, Robert N., and George W. Comstock. "Phlyctenular keratoconjunctivitis among Eskimos in Southwestern Alaska, II: Isoniazid prophylaxis. *American Review of Respiratory Disease* 91 (2): 188–96, February 1965.

Philips, F. J. "A preliminary report of out-patient treatment of pulmonary tuberculosis." *Alaska Medicine* 3: 1–4, March 1961.

Porter, Merilys E., and George W. Comstock. "Ambulatory chemotherapy in Alaska." *Public Health Reports* 77 (12): 1021–32, November 1962.

2. Centers for Disease Control and Prevention (1973–1978)

Barrett, D. H., J. M. Burks, B. McMahon, et al. "Epidemiology of hepatitis B in two Alaska communities." *American Journal of Epidemiology* 105: 118–22, February 1977.

Barrett, D. H., M. S. Eisenberg, T. R. Bender, et al. "Type A and Type B botulism in the North: First reported cases due to toxin other than type E in Alaskan Inuit." *Journal of Adolescent Health Care* 117: 483–89, September 3, 1977.

Blot, W. J., A. Lanier, J. F. Fraumeni Jr., and T. R. Bender. "Cancer mortality among Alaskan Natives, 1960–69." *Journal of the National Cancer Institute* 55: 547–54, September 1975.

Edelen, J. S., T. R. Bender, and T. D. Chin. "Encephalopathy and pericarditis during an outbreak of influenza." *American Journal of Epidemiology* 100: 79–84, August 1974.

Eisenberg, M. S., and T. R. Bender. "Botulism in Alaska, 1947 through 1974: Early detection of cases and investigation of outbreaks as a means of reducing mortality." *Journal of the American Medical Association* 235: 35–38, January 5, 1976.

———. "Plastic bags and botulism: A new twist to an old hazard of the North." *Alaska Medicine* 18: 47–49, July 1976.

Kaplan, G. J., J. K. Fleshman, T. R. Bender, et al. "Long-term effects of otitis media: A ten-year cohort study of Alaskan Eskimo children." *Pediatrics* 52: 577–85, October 1973.

Lanier, A. *Survey of Cancer Incidence in Alaskan Natives.* National Cancer Institute Monograph 47 (1977).

Lanier, A., T. Bender, M. I. Talbot, et al. "Epstein-barr virus DNA in tumour tissue from Native Alaskan patients with nasopharyngeal carcinoma (Letter)." *Lancet* 1095, November 18, 1978.

Lanier, A., T. R. Bender, W. J. Blot, et al. "Cancer incidence in Alaska Natives." *International Journal of Cancer* 18: 409–12, October 15, 1976.

Lanier, A. P., T. R. Bender, C. F. Tschopp, and P. Dohan. "Nasopharyngeal carcinoma in an Alaskan Eskimo family: Report of three cases." *Journal of the National Cancer Institute* 62: 1121–24 May 1979.

Maynard, J. E., D. R. Barrett, B. L. Murphy, et al. "Relation of A antigen to hepatitis B virus infection in an area of hyperendemicity." *Journal of Infectious Diseases* 133: 339–42, March 1976.

Petersen, N. J., D. H. Barrett, W. W. Bond, et al. "Hepatitis B surface antigen in saliva, impetiginous lesions, and the environment in two remote Alaskan villages." *Applied Environmental Microbiology* 32: 572–74, October 1976.

Scott, E. M. "Genetic disorders in isolated populations." *Archives of Environmental Health* 26: 32–35, January 1973.

———. "Genetic diversity of Athabaskan Indians." *Annals of Human Biology* 6: 241–47, May/June 1979.

———. "Inheritance of two types of deficiency of human serum cholinesterase." *Annals of Human Genetics* 37: 139–43, October 1973.

Scott, E. M., and R. C. Wright. "A third type of serum cholinesterase deficiency in Eskimos." *American Journal of Human Genetics* 28: 253–56, May 1976.

———. "Polymorphism of red cell enzymes in Alaskan ethnic groups." *Annals of Human Genetics* 41: 341–46, January 1978.

Index of Proper Names

Page numbers for photographs are in bold type. Agencies and programs of the Public Health Service are listed under "Public Health Service," except for the Centers for Disease Control and Prevention, which has its own entry.

Earle, Bayliss, 44–45, 46
Eastwind, 32
Edwards, Stan, 90, **91**, 134n8
Egg Island, 24, 43, 44
Eisenberg, Mickey S., 68, 131n21
English Bay (Nanwalek), AK, 90, 97
Exxon Valdez, 6
Fairbanks, AK, 4, 11, 54, 56, 60, 78,
131n16; PHS Alaska Native
Health Center at, 105
Farson, Clyde, 105
Federal Employees Compensation
Commission, 40–41
Federal Works Agency, 59
Fellows, Frank, 76–77, 132n19
Fish and Wildlife Service, 94
Fleshman, J. Kenneth, 105
Fort Nelson, BC, Canada, 60; Kehr
General Hospital at, 61
Fort Richardson, AK, 63
Fort St. John, BC, 60
Fort St. Michael, AK, 43
Fort Yukon, AK, 56, 93, 95
Fortuine, Robert, ix, 103, **106**
Foster, Assistant Surgeon, 49
Foster, Milton H., 50, 71–72
Fox, Carroll, 44, 46–48, 70, 128n8
Fox, W. F., 29
Fraser, Robert, 133n6
Galena, AK, 68
Gallagher, Joseph A., 86
Galloway, T. C., Jr., 28–29
Gallup (NM): PHS Indian Medical
Center at, 106
Gardner, C. H., 18, 19, 124n14
Gehrig, Leo, 63–64
Gruening, Ernest, 5, 63, 64, 113
Gulf of Alaska, 14, 15, 19, 35, 47, 52
Haas, Rudolph, 77–78
Haida, 31
Haldeman, Jack C., 110–11, 113,
135n7
Hamilton, John B., 69
Harvard School of Public Health,
117
Hasseltine, H. E., 27, 125n27
Hawley, R. N., 22, 25
Hayes, James, 107
Hays, George A., 62, 63
Health, 81
Healy, Michael, 16–17, 19, 22, 124n9,
124n14
Heimke, David, **106**
Henderson, A. J., 40

Herr, David, **32**
Holland Katherine A., **106**
Hooker, Keith R., 67
Hoonah, AK, 48, 49, 51
Hooper, Calvin L., 16, 38
Horne, Henry, 30
Hospital. *See under geographical
location*
Howard, W. A., 14
Hudson, Charles, 90
Hunter, James A., 86
Hurlburt, Ward, 105
Hygiene, 62, 63, **65**, 66, 81
Hynson, Theodore E., 85, 86
Iditarod Race, 5
Interior Alaska Service Unit, 101
International Boundary Survey, 51
Ivey, Gerald H., 134n20
Jacobsen, Ed, 97
James, William, 105
Japonski Island, 47
Jarvis, D. H., 20–21, 43–45
Jenkins, L. W., 28, 33
Jeraula, F. N. C., 43
Johnson, M. Walter, 104
Jones, T. Stephen, 68
Juneau, AK, 7, 11, 41, 47, 48, 49, 51,
56, 61, 62, 86, 95, 132n16; Alaska
Native Health Service Area
Office at, 84, 85; Bureau of
Education Hospital at, 8, 75, **75**,
76, 78; BIA Area Office at, 76;
BIA Hospital at, 84; PHS Alaska
Native Hospital at, 93; PHS
Alaska Native Health Center at,
94, 95; St. Ann's Hospital at, 36,
37, 95; territorial capital at, 36,
50, 53, 63, 66, 76
Kanakanak, AK, 105, 107; BIA
Hospital at, 9, 84; PHS Alaska
Native Hospital at, 81, 92, 105;
Service Unit, 101
Kasuga, Kazumi, 86, 133n5
Keefer, Jay, **89**
Kehr, Robert W., 60, 61
Ketchikan, AK, 11, 47, 50, 56, 95;
contract services at, 39, 42, 62;
DIH Clinic at, 93, 105; General
Hospital at, 95
Killisnoo, AK, 48, 49
Kinyoun, Joseph, 45
Kiska Island, 5
Klondike, YT, Canada, 4, 11, 46
Kodiak, AK, 28, 40, 41

P 78, 9, 80
P 82

Restaurants